AF841226

## About the Author

Dr William J. Allender is a Forensic Toxicologist and Chartered Chemist (Medicinal Chemistry). He is a qualified expert in drugs, poisons, including pesticides, and alcohol-related matters with over 30 years professional experience. Advises, consults and evaluates matters of forensic concern associated with toxicology of drugs, poisons and alcohol to prosecution, defence and plaintiff lawyers and has provided testimony as an Expert Witness to Courts of law in the states of Australia. He has provided expertise in drug and alcohol related matters including blood and urine drug testing; hair testing; drug facilitated sexual assault; driving under the influence (DUI) cause or contribution to death; cause or contribution of accidents including motor vehicle, hospital, nursing homes and workplace accidents.

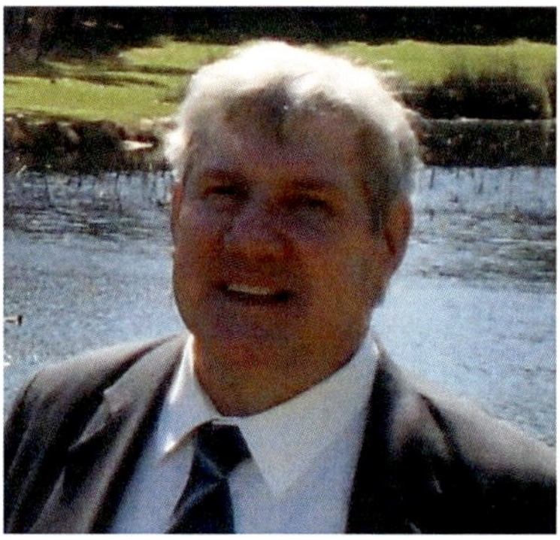

Dr William ("Bill") J. Allender

Forensic Toxicologist/Medical Scientist

## Dedication

Dedicated to the Victims of the Crimes and their Families, the Police Officers and Colleagues I have had the privilege of working with on these, and many other cases.

William J. Allender

# A FORENSIC CASEBOOK

AUSTIN MACAULEY
PUBLISHERS LTD.

A CIP catalogue record for this title is available from the British Library.

ISBN 978 184963 701 5

www.austinmacauley.com

First Published (2014)
Austin Macauley Publishers Ltd.
25 Canada Square
Canary Wharf
London
E14 5LB

Printed and bound in Great Britain

# Contents

# Introduction

I am waiting outside the Coroner's Court at Glebe, Sydney, New South Wales, Australia, to give evidence in yet another case, this one involving another overdose of methadone to a child. The mother is sobbing and grim faces surround her. I think of earlier cases, where a more deliberate approach was adopted to remove someone who was considered 'in the way' or an obstacle. Could this one have been motivated for the same reasons? Some folk are convincing actors…

Poisons and drugs from a variety of sources have been used illegally for centuries and most conjure up an unfortunate, enduring fascination. People appear to be both attracted by them and at the same time repelled by them, due to the fact that they are both deadly and, at the same time, can be very discreet. In forensic investigations, the questions that are usually raised are:

*"Did the victim overdose?*
*"What was the poison/ drug used?"*
*"Was it murder, an accident or suicide?"* and
*"How was it taken and how much?"*

However, the difference may come down to how it was administered, to the probable dosage depending on the potency (a 'touch' maybe too much?), to the levels found in the body, to body weight and to the victim's tolerance, whether or not a regular user of the substance. Then there's always the motive for carrying out the deed.

Here is a selection of cases from the many I have been involved in over the years…

# 1
# Arsenic for Dinner?

*"Selfishness is that detestable vice which no one will forgive in others, and no one is without himself."*

Henry Ward Beecher

**Stake Out**

It was a cool evening in the winter of 1980, and I was sitting in an unmarked police car with two police officers and a detective, outside a block of flats in the suburb of Manly, Sydney, Australia. As the evening wore on, a furtive female figure arrived at the Manly address and unlocked the door to one of the flats. As she went into the flat and turned on the lights, the detective turned and said to me, "Time to go, our quarry has arrived."

With that, three of us got out of the vehicle, while another male police officer stayed with the car. The female police officer that accompanied the detective and I knocked on the door. A middle-aged woman who had clearly seen better days, but was nonetheless smartly dressed, answered the door:

"Yes, what do you want?"

The policewoman replied, "We have a search warrant to search this unit, as we have reasonable suspicion that you have attempted to murder your husband with arsenic."

She then said, "Oh, all right, come on in, I have nothing to hide."

Earlier that day the officer-in-charge (OIC) of the Drug Section at the Division of Analytical Laboratories, Lidcombe (a suburb of Sydney, NSW) was approached by police who asked:

"Do you have someone who can test for arsenic in food?"

I mentioned earlier to the OIC that I had tested for arsenic in the past, and so was nominated for the job....

**Testing, testing...**

Arsenic is usually detected by means of 'Marsh's test'. Arsenic has the distinction of being the first poison for which this diagnostic test was devised. In addition to the suspected material (which maybe food or tissues from the victim) this test involves a small quantity of dilute sulphuric acid followed by the addition of granulated zinc. Acid and zinc alone only produce hydrogen, yet in the presence of arsenic in the test material arsine gas is given off. This gas can be detected by igniting it and holding a piece of glass above the flame. Arsenic is then deposited on the glass as a dark shining "mirror".

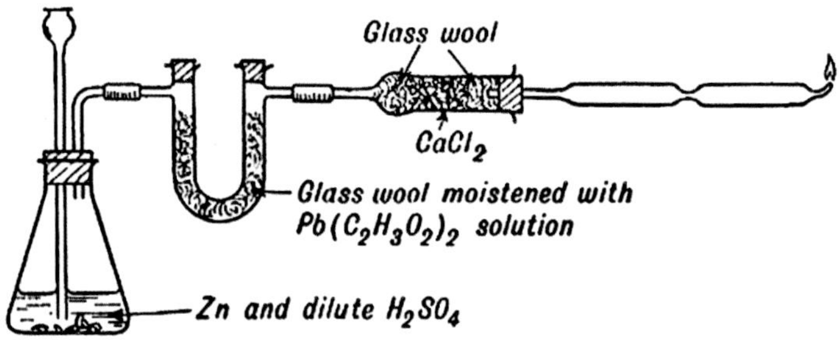


Marsh's Test

Fig. 1 A Test for arsenic

Another test, which is essentially a modification of the Marsh's test, is the 'Gutzeit's test'. The hydrogen is produced as before and the suspected substance added. The gases produced are led up a vertical tube containing rolled-up lead acetate paper, at the end of which is a small sheet of filter paper ( a sort of 'blotting paper') moistened with mercury (mercuric) chloride solution. This is held in position by means of two perforated rubber bungs and a spring clip:

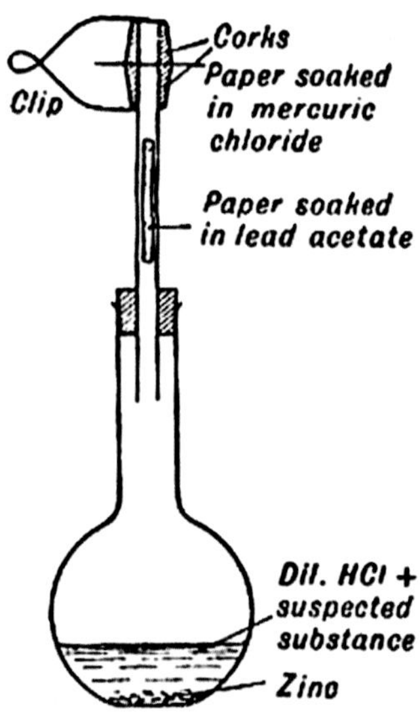


Gutzeit's Test

Fig. 2. Gutzeit's Test for arsenic

If arsenic is present, then the arsine produced stains the mercury chloride paper yellow. The intensity of the yellow-coloured stain produced may be compared to known concentrations of arsenic. The test can then be used for the estimation of the amount of arsenic present. More modern techniques are used now, such as cold vapour atomic fluorescence spectrometry which is highly element-specific. However, at the time I needed a simple, portable kit that could be used in 'the field'.

**So, where was the arsenic?**

I quickly gathered my testing gear. I chose to use the Gutzeit test for arsenic as it provided a colour test and was more specific for arsenic, plus it was possible to roughly determine how much of the toxin was present by comparison to colours generated by known concentrations of arsenic.

The 'kit' consisting of granulated zinc, dilute sulphuric acid and some filter papers previously soaked in mercury chloride – and solutions of arsenic at known concentrations. It was this kit I took to the 'stake out'. An initial test proved positive for a known 'spiked' test sample. Now it was time to test the alleged suspect's samples.

Meanwhile, at the 'stake in' the detective and I were testing numerous foodstuffs, including voluminous amounts of alcohol and food. A check under her bed revealed cases and cases of spirits, wine and beer. Mrs Smith (not her real name) appeared to be stealing liquor from her employer – *big time*! While the testing was being carried out, Mrs Smith was being interviewed by the female police officer in the lounge room of the flat. It appeared that her husband had checked himself into Manly District Hospital and was showing all the signs of arsenic poisoning. In addition, his fingernails and hair were tested for the presence of arsenic – it was positive.

When Mrs Smith was questioned about this, she replied, "I know nothing about this. Our marriage hasn't been very good for some years now, we sleep in separate rooms – but I didn't poison him. Anyway, where would I get the arsenic? I work for a liquor store!!'

Further tests on samples of opened food containers and liquor bottle contents were not showing any positive results. Maybe she was telling the truth… But where was the arsenic?

"She didn't have enough time to flush it down the toilet," commented the detective.

My thoughts exactly… but where was the arsenic stored?

**Back at the laboratory**

Food samples from the refrigerator and an opened bottle of liquor were placed in exhibit bags and transported back to the laboratory for testing and analysis.

Aside from residual (traces of) arsenic in the foodstuffs, certainly not enough to poison a person, the samples did not appear to be a danger to people consuming the food. What now? At that point, I could not contribute any more to the investigation and after I submitted my report, resumed my analyses of illicit drugs casework at the Drug Laboratory at the Division of Analytical Laboratories.

**'Out of the blue'**

It was just over a year later that I again saw the detective about this case.

I asked him out of curiosity, "Well, what happened? Was she [Mrs Smith] charged?

He replied, "It was not her at all. Her husband, who worked in an engineering firm and had access to arsenic, set her up. Arsenic is apparently used to strengthen lead along with other uses. They owned that block of flats they lived in at Manly, and he was not keen to share. So, he poisoned himself with small doses of arsenic, making out it was his wife trying to do him in. He hoped to send her to prison for attempted murder and gain control of a very expensive piece of real estate."

The 'victim' was in fact poisoning himself – albeit at sub-lethal levels!!

I never found out what was the final conclusion to this matter. But what a way to deal with a problem – and it almost succeeded!

# 2
# A Cry in the Night

*"Nobody ever forgets where he buried a hatchet."*

Kin Hubbard

## Introduction

Uralla is a quiet rural town of some 2300 people situated in hilly country on the Northern Tablelands of the New England region of New South Wales. The town is located some twenty-three kilometres south-west of Armidale and 502 kilometres from Sydney.

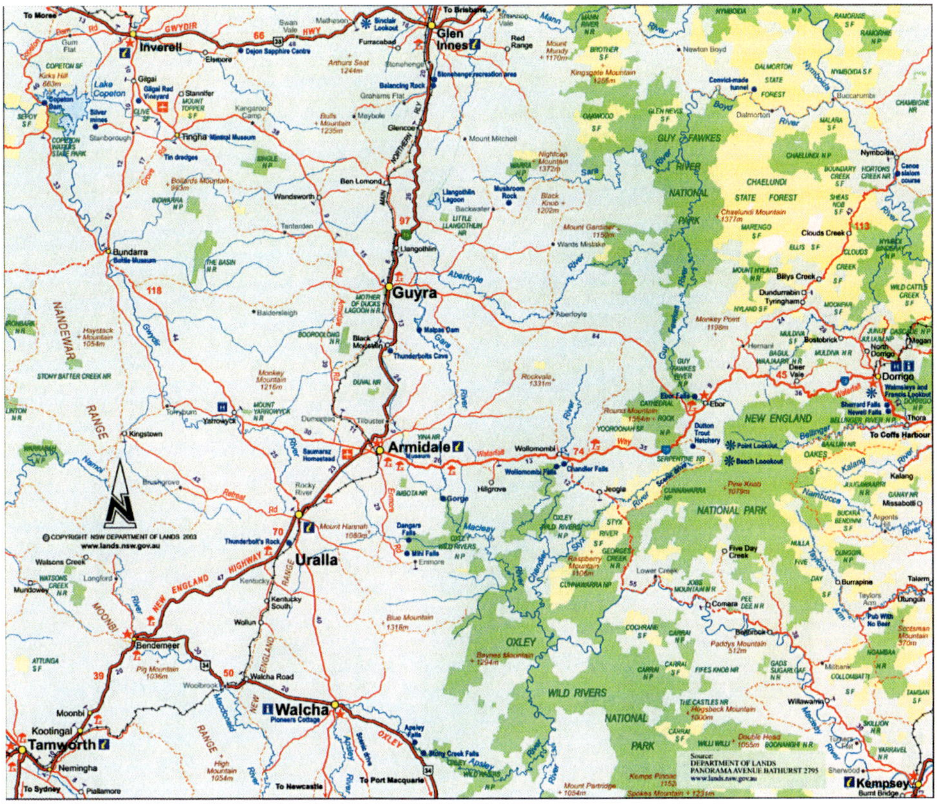


*Fig. 3 Map of New South Wales, Australia showing the location of Uralla.*

The district is renowned for superfine wool and cattle – and the notorious bushranger, Captain Thunderbolt (Fred Ward) who was shot in 1870.

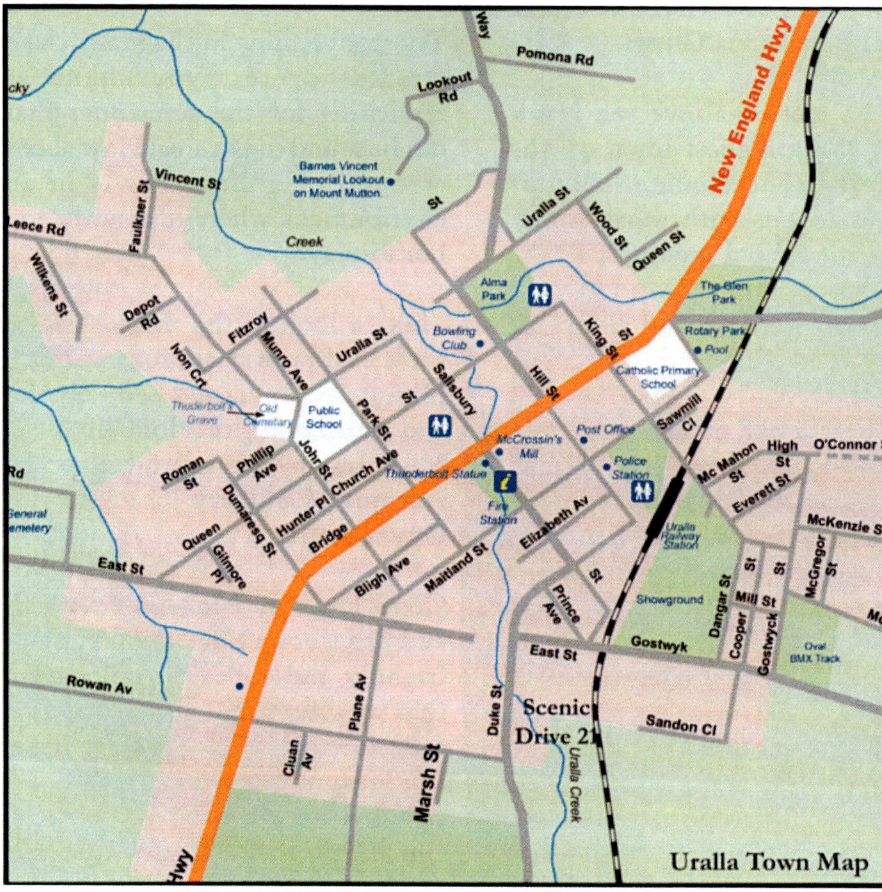


*Fig. 4. A map of Uralla showing Queen Street where the tragedy unfolded.*

However, this quiet village was soon to be disturbed again with a domestic dispute which got way 'out of hand' between two of its residents, Leo ('Snow') Hunt and his de facto wife Marion Reid, which subsequently resulted in her murder at his hands.

## A Troubled Evening

It was a cold, bleak evening in the winter of June 10, 2000, when Uralla Police received a telephone call from a resident at about eight forty p.m. who said, "I am from Queen Street, there is some sort of commotion going on at the flats next door. Could you come and investigate?"

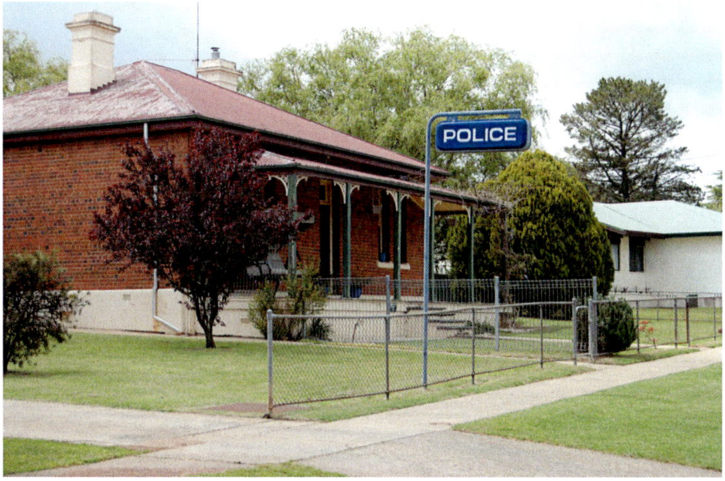


*Fig. 5. Uralla Police Station –*
*Photograph courtesy of Barry Fay, Australian Police Journal*

Police arrived shortly after and found Marion Reid and a young female companion outside a flat. Leo ('Snow') Hunt was standing at the front of the sliding glass door. Marion ('Mary') Reid and Leo ('Snow') Reid had a troubled relationship for some time, which was no doubt worsened by alcohol consumption by both parties. In regard to this, the evening was to prove more troubled than the previous ones. 'Snow' was so known due to his pure white hair and he was part aboriginal – and very possessive and jealous of *his* woman!

Police asked Mary "What's going on Mary?" and she replied, "Snow has assaulted me."

After further discussion it became apparent why this evening was more troubled than others, with this couple, aside from both parties being moderately affected by alcohol.

She said, "Snow is accusing me of having an affair with the bloke in flat four, I don't even know him."

Jealously, coupled with alcohol was clearly playing its part.

Mary was further questioned. "What has happened tonight?"

She said, "He knocked me glasses off me face and forced me up to that bloke's flat, screaming at me." She further reiterated, "He's kicked me and knocked me glasses off me head, I don't even know the bloke in flat four."

The situation was now getting out of hand. 'Snow' lent sideways to Mary and said, "If you get an AVO [Apprehended Violence Order], you're dead, I'll fucking kill you."

Mary Reid then replied, "I didn't get the last AVO, the Police did. I didn't call them tonight."

With that the police officer said, "Get up Snow and wait outside," and "Mary, I'm going to charge him with assault based on what you have told me. I will back in a moment."

An AVO was applied for and subsequently issued by an after-hours magistrate at Parramatta. The terms of this AVO were then read to Hunt.

The police officer then said, "Do you understand all those conditions about not going near Mary?"

Hunt then said, "Yeah, I understand. All this for a fucking gin!"

Unfortunately, Hunt was not locked up at this point, and instead was conditionally bailed not to approach Ms Reid. The time was about eleven fifty-five p.m., and so the tragic event unfolded…

### Misdirected Vengeance

Hunt had no intention of obeying the AVO and planned to carry out his threat, which he subsequently did in the most brutal way. He had to deal with his 'unruly' victim, and evidently reached for a kitchen carving knife to carry it out. What happened next is unclear but the outcome certainly was. 'Snow' apparently went back to Ms Reid's home and somehow coaxed her out of her flat, as the door to her home was not forced even though she was advised by police to, "Lock the door after I [the Police] leave." Unfortunately, it appears Ms Reid did not realise the serious danger she was in, and appears to have opened the door to her aggressor. Then, realising her error, she took off through the caravan park in Uralla chased by Hunt. On catching her, he stabbed her several times in the back, killing her. The knife used in the attack was left embedded in her back.

At about twelve thirty-six a.m. according to witnesses, they heard a woman scream. One who described the sound he heard said, "This scream was like nothing I have ever heard, it was as if this woman was in agony, it was a deep agonising painful scream. It went on for two or three seconds and it stopped for a second and then started again, the same deep painful scream. It went a bit longer than the first scream probably about four seconds and then it went all silent…"

### The Aftermath

At about twelve forty a.m. on Sunday morning 11 June 2000, Police emergency received a triple zero (000) call with the following transcript:

*Transcript of "000" call made on the 11 June, 2000*
*<u>TIME</u> <u>00. 39. 50. 00</u> <u>00. 40. 00</u>*

| | |
|---|---|
| *OPERATOR* | *Hello, emergency. Hello Police emergency.* |
| *CALLER* | *Uralla Police please.* |
| *OPERATOR* | *I can't put you through sir. I can get them to come and see you.* |
| *OPERATOR* | *Hello?* |
| *CALLER* | *I want to speak to Uralla Police please.* |
| *OPERATOR* | *I can't put you through. I can get them to come and see you or I can get them to contact you by phone.* |

| | |
|---|---|
| *CALLER* | *...contact then please* |
| *OPERATOR* | *OK. What's your name?* |
| *CALLER* | *Snow Hunt* |
| *OPERATOR* | *Sorry what was your name sorry?* |
| *CALLER* | *Hunt* |
| *OPERATOR* | *Hunt* |
| *CALLER* | *Xxxxxxx ('phone number given)* |
| *OPERATOR* | *OK. Can I say what it's regarding Mr Hunt?* |
| *CALLER* | *What's that?* |
| *OPERATOR* | *What is it regarding?* |
| *CALLER* | *Oh well I'll talk to the Police.* |
| *OPERATOR* | *OK. You don't have an emergency that you need the Police to attend to straight away?* |
| *CALLER* | *I think so, yes.* |
| *OPERATOR* | *You do need the Police there straight away?* |
| *CALLER* | *Yes, yes please.* |
| *OPERATOR* | *Well it's quicker if you give me the details...* |

*CALL TERMINATED*

At about twelve fifty-five a.m. on Sunday morning 11 June 2000, Uralla Police were contacted and visited 'Snow' Hunt at his residence about ten minutes later.

The house was in darkness and the front door was closed.

However, it opened when Police knocked on it. "Snow are you in there..? What's going on?"

'Snow' slowly emerged from the darkness and replied, "What..?"

Uralla Police further questioned, "What's going on, why did you call the cops talking about Mary?"

He replied, "You obviously don't know what's happened."

Hunt was further asked several times, "Where's Mary?"

Eventually he answered, "In the park."

Constable Styles then asked, "Where in the park?"

Hunt replied, "In the caravan park."

Constable Styles, "What have you done to her?"

After some further discussion Hunt led the Police to the scene of the crime, and as he pointed towards a body lying in the grass, said, "There she is."

Ms Mary Reid was found lying face down in the grass of the Uralla Caravan Park, with a large amount of blood around her nose and mouth area. A large-handled kitchen knife used in the attack was still embedded in her back.

Hunt was further asked by Police, "What have you done?" This was in reference to the deceased. However, Hunt surprisingly said, "I have had two packets of Serepax and I don't know what I've done." He was questioned about the origin of the knife and said, "What knife? I don't know."

Hunt was then placed under arrest and cautioned.

A short time later further Police and an ambulance arrived at the crime scene. An ambulance officer checked the deceased for any signs of life, who was also asked, "Can you check the prisoner? He said that he has taken two packets of Serepax." Police that had arrived advised, "They will need to take him to hospital. Get him out and handcuff him." Hunt was handcuffed and then escorted by police to the ambulance, which left a short time later for Armidale Hospital.

In the meantime the crime scene was preserved until crime scene and detective police arrived. A search was made of 'Snow' Hunt's premises where two empty blister packs bearing the logo 'Serepax' were found. A Government contractor arrived at about seven thirty a.m. at the Uralla Caravan Park and took MsReid's body to Armidale Hospital, where her life was pronounced extinct by a resident doctor, then conveyed to the mortuary.

**Hunt at the Hospital**

The ambulance transported 'Snow' Hunt to the Accident and Emergency Section arriving at one fifty-seven a.m.

On the way Hunt appeared "alert and orientated and there were no other complaints." The doctor on duty was briefed on what happened.

Hunt was asked, "What happened?" and he replied, "I warned her…"

The nursing staff commenced to hook Hunt up to a monitor that checked his cardiac and respiratory systems, while carrying out these duties the police officer was asked if the handcuffs were really necessary. It was at this stage that nursing staff were told that Hunt was alleged to have murdered someone earlier in the evening and that he had taken two foil packs of Serepax (a brand of oxazepam). Part of the treatment for the drug overdose was to administer charcoal to absorb any of the poisons. Hunt was unhappy with this procedure and said, "Do I have to have this shit?" The treating nurse simply said, "Sorry, you have to have it."

Further tests were conducted including a Glascow coma test. This is to determine how alert a person is, 15 is totally normal. Hunt was assessed as 14.

"The only area that Mr Hunt seemed confused on was where he was," reported one medic.

Clearly, the amount of oxazepam he had apparently ingested was having a minimal effect at this stage. He was asked by nursing staff, "What have you taken?"

Hunt replied, "Two packets of Serepax." At this time he smelt strongly of alcohol.

At for thirty a.m. a Glascow test was again performed on Hunt by nursing staff and there was no response to speech or spontaneous action. However, after a final test involving a sternal rub, Hunt awoke and started to throw his arms around and swinging punches at nursing staff. Given his behaviour, he had to be restrained and so was handcuffed again. During this time he was abusing at everyone and was saying things such as, "What the fuck are you doing?"

At six a.m. a further Glascow test was carried out and now he only rated 10, and only responded to the sternal rub. So the handcuff was undone and, as nursing staff attempted to aid his respiration, he suddenly propped himself up on his elbow and said, "I'm going to kill you."

He took a swing at the attending nurse who screamed, further staff came to her aid and so the handcuffs were returned in order to restrain him. Eventually, he settled at seven a.m. Clearly, Hunt had developed a tolerance to the drug oxazepam, and he had apparently been taking the drug for many years to 'settle him down'. Any alcohol present would have exacerbated the effects.

### Drug Levels Found in Hunt's Blood

A blood sample taken from Hunt at the Armidale Hospital at twelve noon that day was found to contain oxazepam 2.2 milligrams per litre (mg/L). I found the level of oxazepam in his blood was particularly high and was over eight times the therapeutic range (0.09 to 0.44 mg/L, average 0.265 mg/L).

No alcohol was recorded in the blood sample. Though a witness said, "He smelt strongly of alcohol and I would say he was about half drunk. Snowy was talking normally and he was having no trouble standing up or walking."

However, given the time interval, it is more probable that any alcohol had been metabolised (digested) to undetectable levels. Also, 'Snow' being a regular drinker of alcohol would be more tolerant of liquor and able to metabolise it faster than an irregular or social consumer of alcohol.

### Postmortem of Victim

The post mortem of Mary Reid's body showed that she appeared to have had a rough life prior to her death, with a number of bruises of varying ages covering her body and several health problems being revealed. More importantly, she clearly died a terrible death from the several stabbing blows delivered by her murderer. The wounds that most likely took her life were apparent in her chest. Defensive injuries to her hands showed she had desperately tried to prevent her life from being taken from her. And the final indignity, the kitchen knife that was used in the murderous attack was then left imbedded in her back.

### On Trial for Murder

On 12 November, 2001 Leo ('Snow') Vincent Hunt, stood trial in the NSW Supreme Court at Tamworth for murder (1) of Marion Louise Reid on 11 June, 2000.

I attended Tamworth Court for the committal hearing, and gave evidence as to the level of drug, oxazepam found in Hunt's blood. I was cross examined on a number of issues relating to the drug, including time of absorption, quantities, time of onset of effects, tolerance etc. For example, "If something of the order of fifty Serepax tablets were taken at one sitting, how would that manifest itself in the stomach, those fofty tablets?

I replied, "Well taking such a large amount it'd form basically what you might call a bolus, that's basically the tablets are clumped together in the stomach and then it's absorbed over a period of time, depending whether food was present."

Further questions, included the possibility that oxazepam ingestion can produce a paradoxical reaction of 'acute rage' rather than sedation, were put to me including, "So from what you know of this case, and based on your knowledge generally, there's nothing that makes it impossible, if one of these paradoxical reactions, acute rage, stimulation or excitement, were to occur? There's nothing that would make it impossible for that to occur within, say, fifteen minutes of a large overdose of tablets having been taken? I mean you can't rule that out, is what I'm putting to you?

I replied, 'Fifteen minutes seems a bit too fast for me. It would have to be at least a minimum of half an hour. You've to allow time for the stomach to actually absorb the drug into the bloodstream, you would be still looking at half an hour to an hour for the effects to actually to come into play [effect]."

Essentially what was being sought from both parties was the anser to the question, Did Hunt take the drug overdose before the murder or after? It seemed more likely the drug overdose was taken *after* the murder, possibly in an attempt to take his own life as well. However, even if the drug overdose was taken just *before* the murder (and there seems to be no motivation to do this) there was insufficient time for the drug to manifest the various effects put to me, paradoxical or otherwise. These were no doubt borne out by other witnesses' evidence that followed my toxicological evidence.

**Conclusion**

The cruel vengeance attack was truly pointless. 'Snow' Hunt had threatened her about an AVO, which she had ***not*** implemented – and he still attacked her, with fatal consequences. The jury and judge apparently felt the same. He was found guilty as charged, and sentenced to a minimum of twenty years imprisonment. Given that 'Snow' was sixty-eight years old at the time of sentencing, he may well spend the remains of his life in gaol. But some folk in Uralla will always remember Mary's agonising cry in the night, when she lost her life in a fit of jealously and rage from a former 'lover'..!

# 3
# A Case of MDMA Madness

*"No one other than you yourself is*
*the cause of your ecstasy or agony."*

Sumit

## Introduction

MDMA (or 3,4 – methylenedioxymethamphetamine) is a popular drug of abuse. Its subjective effects have contributed to its popularity as a 'party drug' among adolescents and young adults, who attend 'rave' or rock parties. This drug is commonly known as Ecstasy and from time to time features in the media.

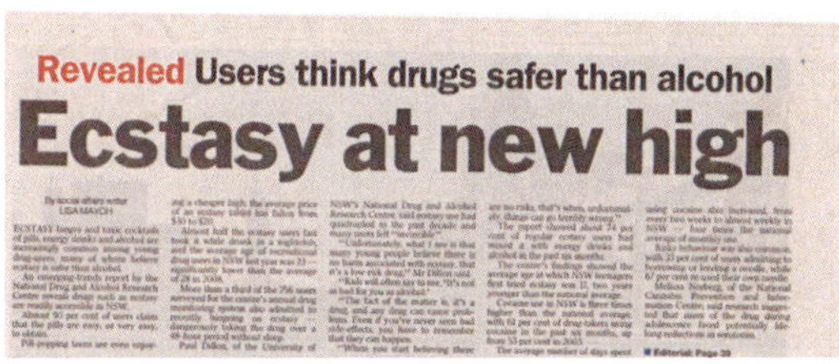
Revealed Users think drugs safer than alcohol

Ecstasy at new high

*Fig. 7. A typical headline-*
*Source:* Daily Telegraph.

The majority of the drug is smuggled into Australia, although there have been some local attempts to synthesise the drug. Unfortunately, the 'local product' is gaining popularity…

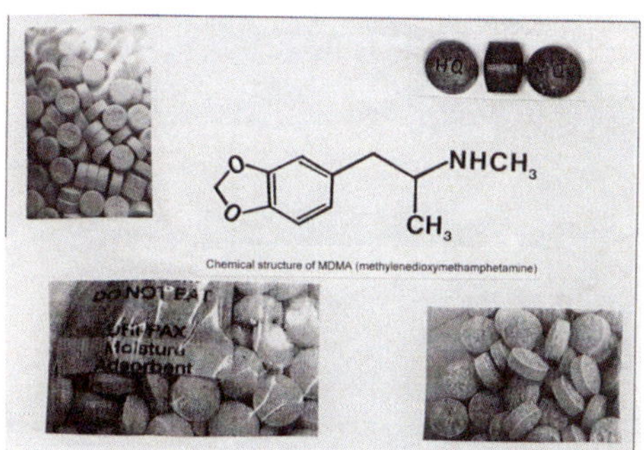


*Fig. 8. Chemical structure of the MDMA and some dosage forms*

MDMA is a ring-substituted derivative of phenethylamine, which has close structural features related to both amphetamines and hallucinogens, such as mescaline. MDMA is used recreationally for its combination of stimulant and hallucinogenic effects, which combines the effects of mescaline and amphetamine. The drug has no approved medical use in Australia but is widely abused. Other 'street names' used for MDMA include: *XTC. Vitamin E* and

*ADAM.* Common methods of taking MDMA include: orally (generally in tablet form), 'snorting' (absorbed nasally), injecting intra-venously and by suppositories.

MDMA is rapidly absorbed when taken orally (the usual method of ingestion) but 'snorting', injecting and suppositories were also reported as methods of ingesting the drug. Injecting has been reported as having the quickest onset and producing a more intense but shorter lasting experience. The effect of taking larger doses was reported as mainly hallucinatory with increased undesirable side effects as the dose is increased. The onset of action is usually within thirty-to-forty minutes and a maximal response is achieved in about one or two hours. The duration of action is about four to six hours (average five hours) and the drug and its metabolites are excreted, mainly in the urine.

The negative effects of Ecstasy are *dose-related*, in that their severity correlates with both the total number of doses consumed and the *frequency of use.* Short-term high dose use of MDMA has produced incidences of an amphetamine-like psychosis and, in some cases, severe hyperthermia that was unresponsive to medical intervention leading to death. It can also cause a paranoid psychosis or chemically induced 'madness'.

One such case occurred early in the morning of 27 January, 2001 when an MDMA-intoxicated man of twenty-three was involved in a fatal motor vehicle collision whilst struggling with police, in the southbound lanes of the Sydney Harbour Bridge.

**The 'Big Day Out'**

It seems prior to the incident that he had attended the "Big Day Out" (or BDO) on the 26 January, 2001.

The BDO began in 1992 and is now the longest-running and biggest rock festival in Australia. Its travelling circus of nearly 100 local and international acts play in five Australian cities and Auckland (New Zealand) to a total audience of about 200,000, making it one of the biggest in the world. In Sydney, the BDO drew a crowd of 55,000 music fans who sweated to the sounds of Australia's biggest band, Powder Finger, Germany's fire-breathing Rammstein, the headline act Limp Bizkit and five separate rooms of disc jockeys.

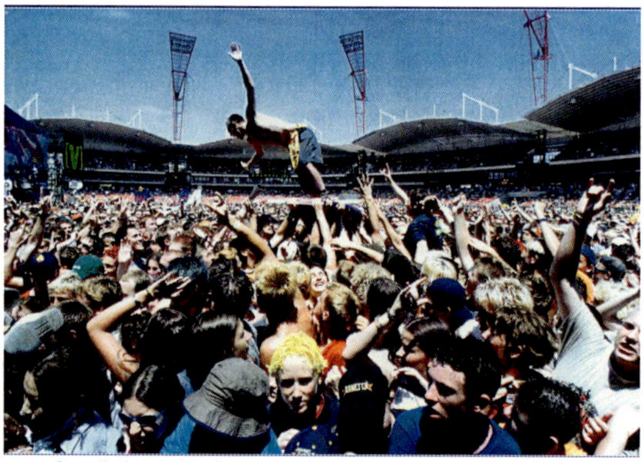

*Fig. 9. Photograph of the BDO crowd - Courtesy of* Sydney Morning Herald.

It appears he purchased the drug during the concert, and at the conclusion of the BDO, went to a friend's house at Neutral Bay, Sydney. It seems that it was his intention to sleep at this residence and return home the following morning. This was ascertained from a mobile phone text message that was sent to his girlfriend at one thirty-four a.m.: "Hi, I'm at Jeb's house in Neutral Bay. I'll be back either early or late, say nineish."

However, at approximately two thirty a.m. he left the premises at Neutral Bay, and his whereabouts at this time are unknown. At approximately four a.m., a male friend contacted him on his mobile phone, only to receive a tirade of abuse and hang up. Further attempts to contact him failed, until about four thirty a.m., when he told them that he was on the Sydney Harbour Bridge. His friend further commented that he had, "Turned funny all of a sudden."

**'King of the Bridge'**

Police subsequently received numerous complaints from motorists reporting a young man walking down the middle of the Harbour Bridge. From some reports he had been attempting to jump in front of the motor vehicles, in an attempt to make them collide with him. In one instance, he reportedly jumped onto a car and was kicking and punching the vehicle.

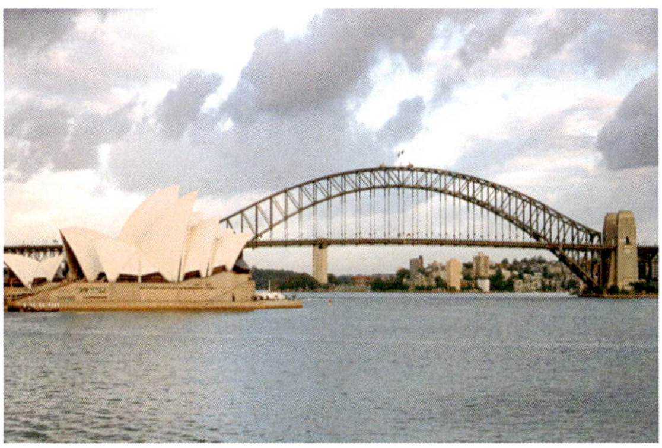

*Fig. 10. Sydney Harbour Bridge on the day of the incident.*

Police arrived on the Sydney Harbour Bridge at about five twenty-five a.m. and attempted to remove him from the Bridge, by placing him in the rear of the Police truck. On being escorted to the truck, he began struggling with police, and eventually kicked off the side of the truck, resulting in all parties falling to the roadway. After this he was sprayed with capsicum spray with no apparent effect. A short time later, a motor vehicle driven south narrowly avoided striking the police, but struck the young man who sustained very serious injuries.

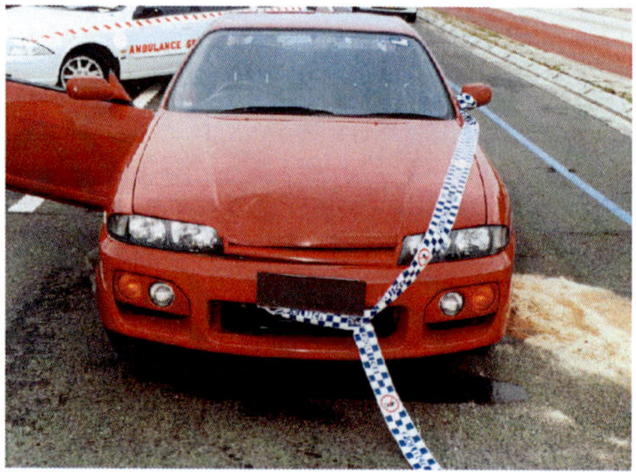

*Fig. 11. Photograph of vehicle which struck the victim*

An ambulance and paramedics arrived at the scene, but the injuries he sustained in the accident were too great to support life. He was later pronounced deceased.

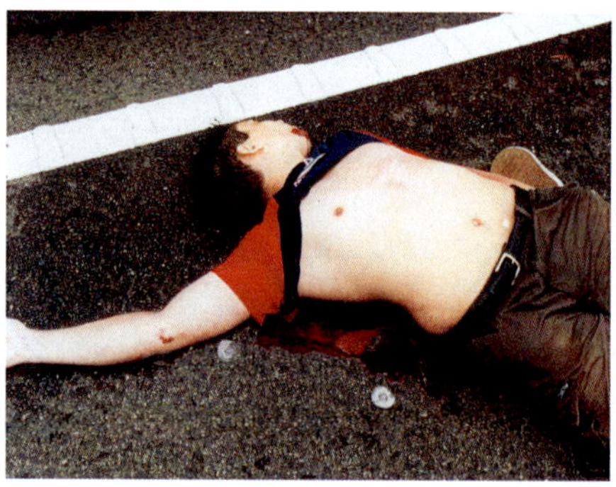

*Fig. 12.*

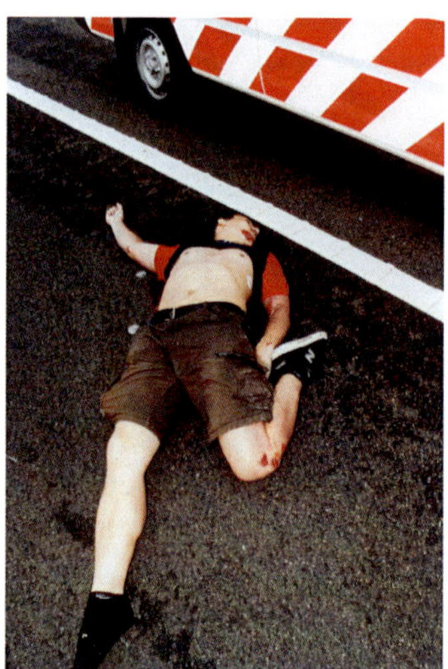

*Figs. 12. & 13. Photographs of the deceased*

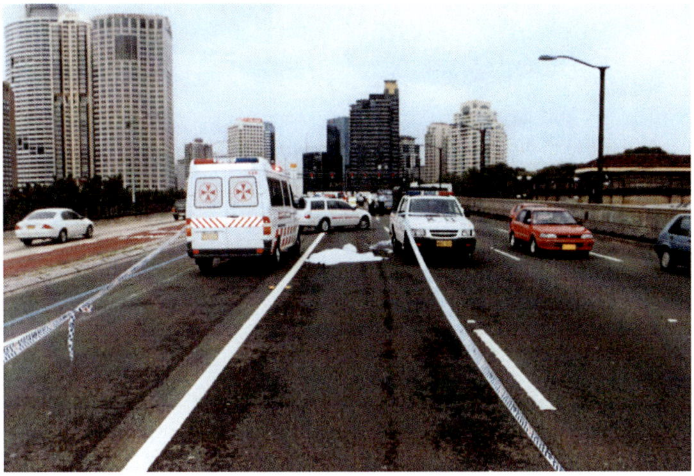

*Fig. 14. Ambulance and paramedics (view south of Sydney Harbour Bridge)*

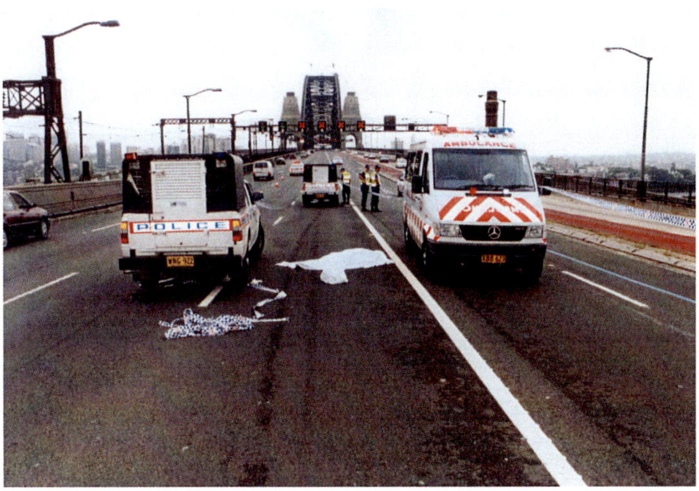


*Fig. 15. Ambulance and paramedics (view north of Sydney Harbour Bridge)*
*[Photographs: NSW Police Crime Scene]*

**Blood Levels Found**

A blood sample taken from the deceased at autopsy was found to contain MDMA 2.1 milligrams per litre and methamphetamine 0.3 milligrams per litre.

I found the level of MDMA in his blood was particularly high and was well within the lethal range, which I later reiterated at the Coroner's Court.

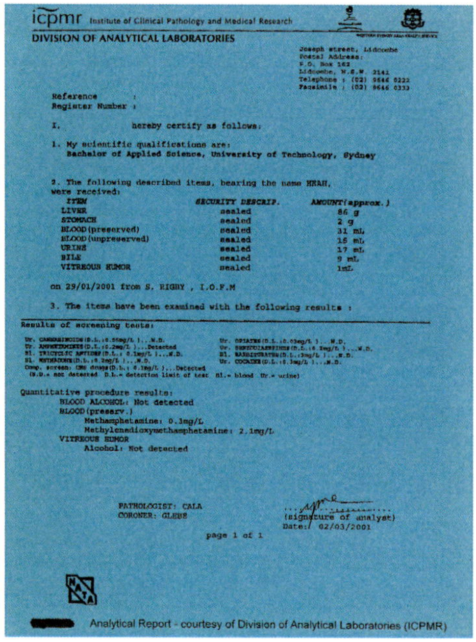

icpmr Institute of Clinical Pathology and Medical Research

DIVISION OF ANALYTICAL LABORATORIES

Joseph street, Lidcombe
Postal Address:
P.O. Box 162
Lidcombe, N.S.W. 2141
Telephone : (02) 9646 0222
Facsimile : (02) 9646 0333

Reference :
Register Number :

I, hereby certify as follows:

1. My scientific qualifications are:
Bachelor of Applied Science, University of Technology, Sydney

2. The following described items, bearing the name HRAH, were received:

| ITEM | SECURITY DESCRIP. | AMOUNT(approx.) |
|---|---|---|
| LIVER | sealed | 86 g |
| STOMACH | sealed | 2 g |
| BLOOD(preserved) | sealed | 31 mL |
| BLOOD(unpreserved) | sealed | 16 mL |
| URINE | sealed | 17 mL |
| BILE | sealed | 9 mL |
| VITREOUS HUMOR | sealed | 1mL |

on 29/01/2001 from S. RIGBY , I.O.F.M

3. The items have been examined with the following results :

Results of screening tests:

Ur. CANNABINOIDS(D.L.:0.05mg/L )...N.D.
Ur. AMPHETAMINES(D.L.:0.2mg/L )...Detected
Bl. TRICYCLIC ANTIDEP(D.L.: 0.1mg/L )...N.D.
Bl. METHADONE(D.L.:0.2mg/L )...N.D.
Comp. screen: CNS drugs(D.L.: 0.1mg/L )...Detected
Ur. OPIATES(D.L.:0.03mg/L )...N.D.
Ur. BENZODIAZEPINES(D.L.:0.1mg/L )...N.D.
Bl. BARBITURATES(D.L.:3mg/L )...N.D.
Ur. COCAINE(D.L.:0.3mg/L )...N.D.
(N.D.= not detected D.L.= detection limit of test Bl.= blood Ur.= urine)

Quantitative procedure results:
BLOOD ALCOHOL: Not detected
BLOOD(preserv.)
Methamphetamine: 0.3mg/L
Methylenedioxymethamphetamine: 2.1mg/L
VITREOUS HUMOR
Alcohol: Not detected

PATHOLOGIST: CALA
CORONER: GLEBE

(signature of analyst)
Date: 02/03/2001

page 1 of 1

NATA

[redacted] Analytical Report - courtesy of Division of Analytical Laboratories (ICPMR)

*Fig. 16. Analyst's Report [Division of Analytical Laboratories, Lidcombe, NSW.]*

This indicated a very high dosage (estimated at approximately 1 gram of the pure drug ingested orally) and suggests that the deceased was a heavy user of MDMA. Whether this was true or not, I was unable to ascertain, but certainly indicated a large dosage had been ingested. I suggested that the presence of the methamphetamine may have been due to either direct ingestion of methamphetamine or that the methamphetamine may have been present in the original MDMA preparation.

MDMA and its congeners constitute potential health hazards of uncertain proportions for human users. Behavioural manifestations of MDMA use by the deceased prior to his death were typical and distinctive. They included rapid and confused speech, dilated pupils, agitation, paranoia and violent, aggressive demeanour. The degree of the effects present generally increased with the blood MDMA concentration, with the violent, paranoid behaviour being attributed to the very high blood MDMA concentration.

## The Inquest

The inquest took place on 21 November, 2001 and it was obvious from the outset that he was a popular, much loved young man, as friends and family members openly wept during proceedings, at one time necessitating a brief adjournment so they could compose themselves…

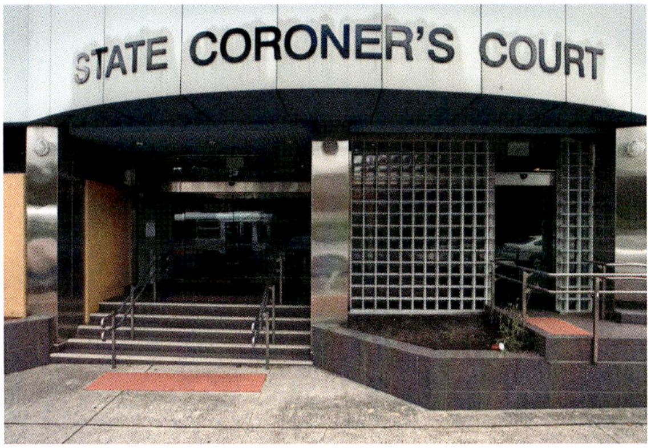


*Fig. 17. Coroner's Court – outside the building on Parramatta Road, Sydney, NSW.*

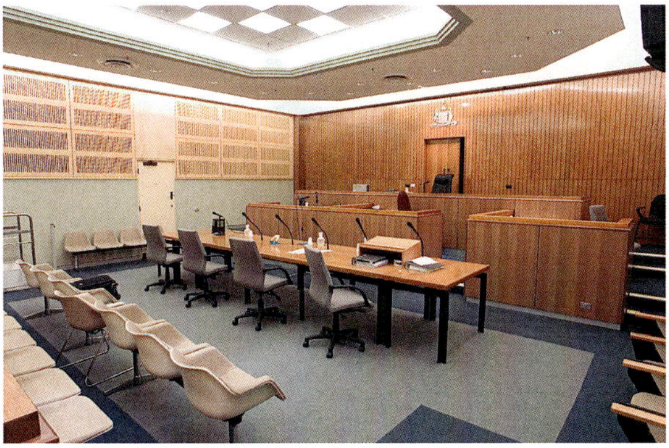

*Fig. 18. Coroner's Court – inside the building*

I took to the witness box and said much of what I said earlier. This was supported by a brief from Professor Graham Starmer, then with the Department of Pharmacology, Sydney University.

It was clear that his bizarre behaviour exhibited on the Harbour Bridge was much out of character, and was almost certainly attributed to the effects of very large doses of MDMA and methamphetamine. Whether these drugs were mixed together, or one was an impurity, is not known.

## Conclusion

It should be noted that the post-mortem blood levels obtained for either drug were potentially lethal. Moreso the MDMA level, and therefore the collision may have simply hastened the final outcome. However, given the level of the drugs detected, if given rapid medical intervention, he may have survived, but we will never know.

# 4
# Affairs of the Heart and Poisons

*"If you drink from a bottle marked 'Poison'*
*you are bound to suffer."*

Lewis Carroll, *Alice through the Looking Glass.*

## Introduction

Most of the poisoning cases I have become involved with and provided Expert advice/evidence at local, district and Supreme Court levels were mostly the more common drugs such as the stimulants, for example: MDMA or Ecstasy, methamphetamine, amphetamine, ephedrine, phentermine, the central nervous system (CNS) depressants such as morphine, heroin, benzodiazepines (eg. diazepam, oxazepam etc.), cannabis, methadone and of course, alcohol.

However, from time to time unusual poisons have appeared in my casework. Two such cases involving pesticides rather than drugs, and are described as follows.

## 1. The Grieving Greenkeeper

A twenty-one-year-old man employed as a greenkeeper developed an infatuation for a pretty young woman. Unfortunately, it was a case of unrequited love, and he became deeply depressed and spoke of suicide. His last words to fellow work mates were, "I just can't live without her…"

Sometime later, he was found by a fellow worker in a semi-conscious state lying on his stomach behind the greenkeeper's shed. The young man had been vomiting after apparently swallowing a quantity of herbicide mixture prior to being found. A container marked 'Endothal' herbicide was found alongside his body. An ambulance was called and he was quickly taken to a nearby hospital where, unfortunately, he died two hours later.

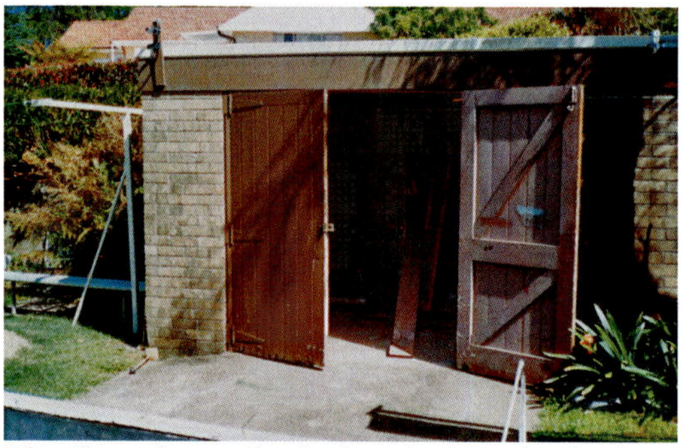

*Fig. 19. The Greenkeeper's shed and where his body was found.*

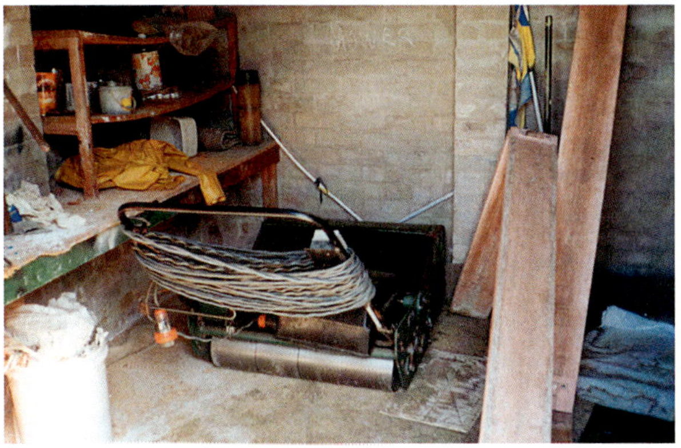

*Fig. 20. Inside the greenkeeper's shed with a variety of lawn chemicals.*

## The Post Mortem

The deceased was a well-developed young male Caucasian weighing 54 kilograms and 1.7 metres tall. The post mortem revealed widespread focal haemorrhages and oedema in his lungs. His gastrointestinal tract showed gross haemorrhage, and his stomach contained a quantity of heavily bloodstained fluid – clearly, he had had a painful death. Curiously, there was blistering around his mouth which I had not expected, given the type of the herbicide consumed.

## The Herbicide

Endothal is used as a selective herbicide, generally in the form of the disodium salt. The herbicide is used for selective control of weed in couch, bent and buffalo grass lawns. It is also used for the defoliation of cotton (prior to harvesting) and for control of aquatic weeds and algae. The product is considered moderately toxic. It is possible that humans may be more susceptible to this substance, as sodium endothal when fed to rats at a concentration of 1000 parts per million (ppm) causes no ill effects, whilst in humans "ingestion may cause vomiting, diarrhea."[diarrhoea].

## Structural Change

Whilst endothal is stable to light, it is readily converted to anhydride, a substance known as norcantharidin at temperatures above ninety degrees centigrade. Whilst summer temperatures in the greenkeeper's shed would soar to the mid-forties and maybe higher, a temperature 'hike' of this magnitude in a stored can seemed impossible to imagine. Although the can may have been stored inadvertently near a heater in winter. However, the can may have been left outside in the sun, resulting in elevated temperatures within the can during summer applications.

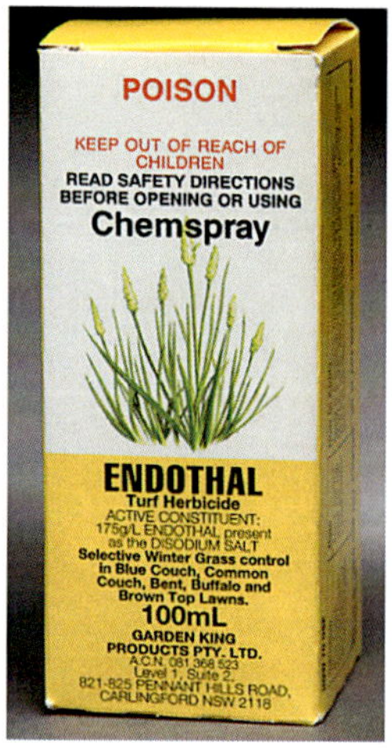


*Fig. 21. A typical pack containing the herbicide, endothal.*

However, the storage conditions of the can are unknown. In any case, a chemical analysis revealed the presence of a small amount of norcantharidin in the formulation. Norcantharidin is very similar in structure to cantharidin.

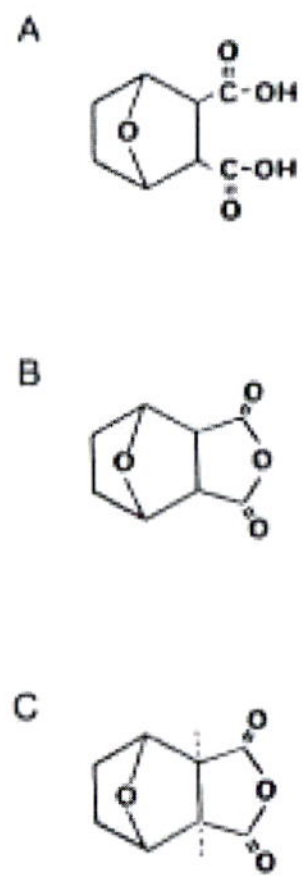


*Fig. 22. Chemical structures of (A) endothall, (B) cantharidin and (C) norcantharidin*

Cantharidin is the active principle of *cantharides* or blister beetles of which the best known is the 'Spanish fly'. This insect is not a 'fly' but an emerald-coloured beetle. Cantharidin is a toxic, irritant chemical. It causes blisters and was formerly used in veterinary medicine as a vesicant, a counterirritant and also as an aphrodisiac (for humans – and surprisingly, also for the beetles!)

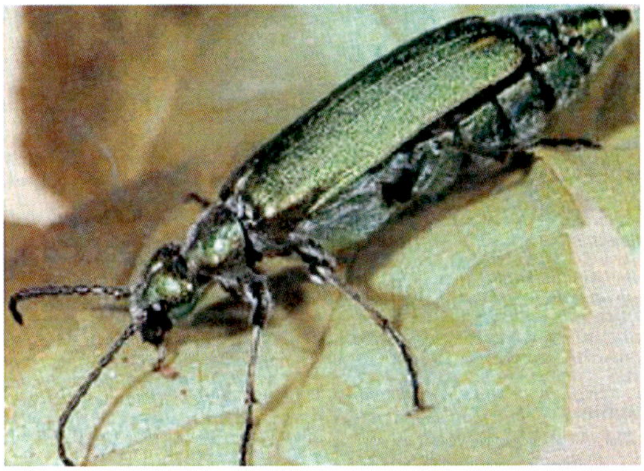

*Fig. 23. Blister beetle or 'Spanish fly'*

However, a dose of only 30 milligrams and as little as 10 milligrams (about as much that can be placed on a match head) has proven fatal in humans.

**Coronial Finding**

The coronial finding was death from suicide from an irritant, corrosive substance. Norcatharidin was found to be a contaminant in the herbicide preparation and was possibly a contributing factor to the greenkeeper's untimely death…

**2. The Vengeful Farmer**

A married couple in the country were having marital problems. The bored farmer's wife was having a number of affairs. As in small country towns, word soon reached her husband and unbeknown to her, the husband had discovered a more recent liaison. He plotted to murder her…

**The Plan**

He had used 'Phosdrin' in the past to kill foxes, so that should do the job! On 20 May, 2001 the Police were called to the farm after it was alleged that the farmer had poisoned his wife with Phosdrin. He had apparently added "half a mil [millilitre] of Phosdrin to her medication of Colloidal Silver" which she took on a daily basis. His wife was into 'natural therapy' products, a form of homeotherapy, and apparently 'Colloidal Silver' was believed to be a naturopathic treatment for asthma.

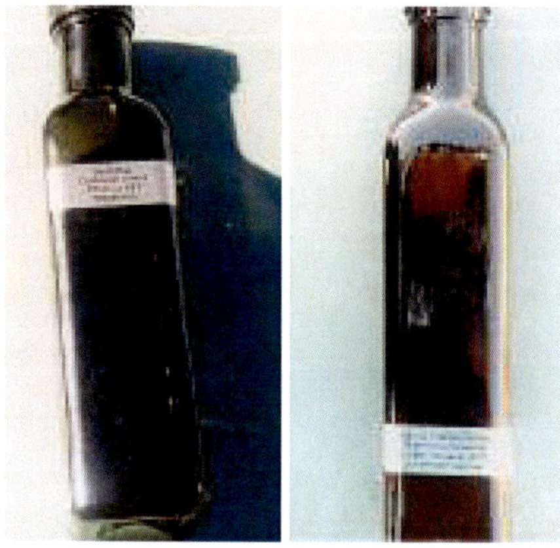

*Fig. 24. Two views of the bottle of "colloidal silver" used by the victim.*

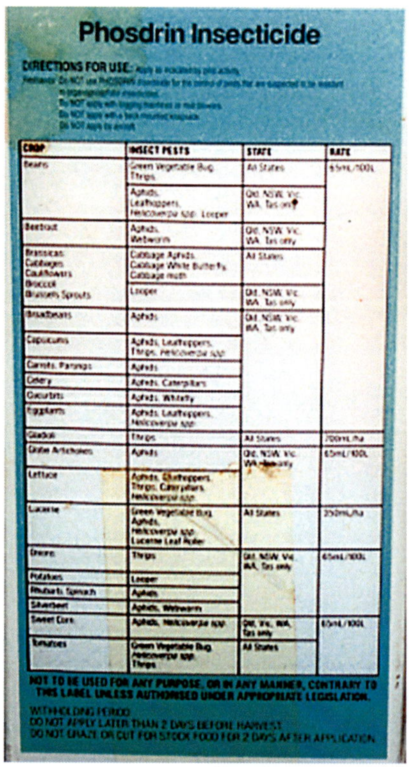


*Fig. 25.Phosdrin label from pack used in the attempted murder.*

On the morning of the offence, the wife said that she had "tasted and swallowed a little bit." The foul taste encountered caused her to spit out and rinse her mouth with water.

Later she stated that she "felt quite woozy, not able to focus properly" and "was shaking violently", had "no control over my bowels" and "threw up violently all over the floor in the toilet."

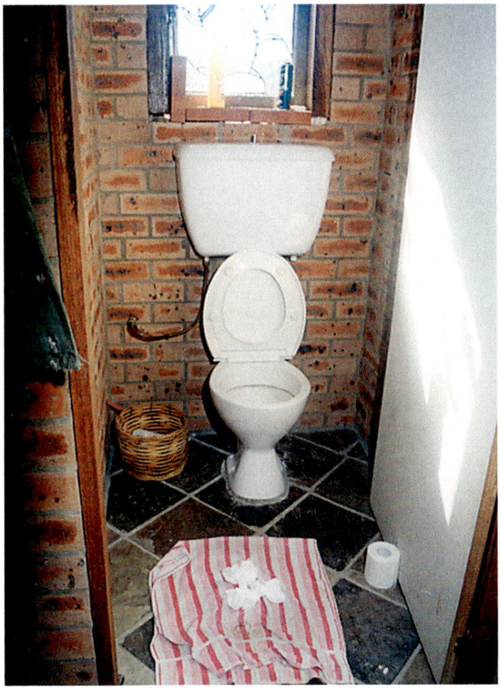

*Fig. 26. Mevinphos or Phosdrin was detected in the vomitus-stained towel lying on the toilet floor.*

An ambulance was called and she was found sitting in a chair, sobbing. An officer said to her, "What happened?" and she said, "My husband's poisoned me." She was treated at hospital, where fortunately she recovered, as it appeared that the bulk of the poison was removed from her body through spitting it out and subsequent vomiting.

**The Analyst's Findings**

A blood sample taken from the wife that day was examined for the presence of mevinphos, and none was detected. A bottle of red liquid marked 'Phosdrin' was found to contain mevinphos, as was the 'AHIMSA Colloidal Silver' medication. Mevinphos was also detected in a drinking glass, and in the vomitus-stained towel taken from the toilet.

## The Poison

Mevinphos is a highly toxic organophosphorus insecticide which is toxic through all routes of exposure, including ingestion, skin absorption and inhalation. Poisoning affects the central nervous system and the eyes. Its toxic action is direct and quick, regardless of the route of exposure. Toxic effects include nausea, vomiting, diarrhoea, abdominal cramps, headache, dizziness, blurred vision, salivation, sweating and confusion. These symptoms of poisoning have appeared in humans within as little as *fifteen minutes* or *as long as two hours* after exposure to mevinphos.

## The Trial

The husband was initially charged with attempted murder. When the matter went to trial, and after some legal wrangling, the charge was reduced to "Administer poison with intent to injure." However, the wife proved to be the defence's best witness by changing her evidence or, in Police terminology, 'doing a back flip' in the witness box!

[This conjures up a rather tricky athletic manoeuvre! However, it means a witness totally changes their evidence sometimes the complete opposite to that previously given].

The evidence from the victim went more or less like this, "and then I realised he only did it... I felt that he only did it to frighten me. He could, he could probably cut my throat, or he could have given me a whole heap, and given me a cup of tea. Phosdrin works within three seconds."

[Note: Not even deadly cyanide works this fast!]

Unfortunately, I was not called to give expert testimony and let the Court know just how close to death she had come. But for her rapid bodily functions removing the bulk of the poison, the outcome may have been quite different. Mevinphos is a very potent poison and, to put it in perspective, was developed from a nerve gas programme during the Second World War. This substance and its close cousins (various chemical analogues) were designed to kill – and kill effectively!

## The Outcome

I spoke to the Department of Public Prosecutions (DPP) and asked what likely sentence would have been appropriate for an offence of this nature, and they indicated at least a period of "penal servitude". The defendant was only sentenced to "250 hours of community service" but no "penal servitude". Not bad for what, in my opinion, amounted to attempted murder...

# 5
# The Corpse in the Culvert

*"The darkness of the soul is not lighted by moving the body to another place."*

Eastern Proverb

## Introduction

Wollongong is an industrial town of over 250,000 people situated in picturesque South Coast of New South Wales. The town is located just over eighty-four kilometres from Sydney and is noted for its iron and steel production at Port Kembla – and its beautiful beaches and the escarpment semi-rainforest. Unfortunately, the 'dark side' of human nature can occur anywhere. This case involved the use of the drug, LSD (lysergic acid diethylamide) along with the consumption of liberal quantities of alcohol, at a local tavern by the participants of this crime.

LSD was really a drug of the past, the 'hippie' 60s and 70s generation where its allegedly carefree properties were promoted by Dr Timothy Leary in the late 60s with the manta 'turn on, tune in, and drop out' (of society). This supposedly 'something snappy' phrase was used to promote the so-called 'benefits' of LSD. Unfortunately, the reverse was true, the drug upsets the brain chemistry of the user resulting in hallucinogens and various other behavioural problems – with the dreaded 'flashbacks' which occur without the drug even being detected in the bloodstream. In fact, LSD is one of the most potent hallucinogenic drugs known, and yet it has a remarkably low acute toxicity, with a therapeutic index (therapeutic ratio) being in the order of 1000. The therapeutic index is a rough indication of how safe a drug is likely to be – the higher the better. However, in practise, this is quite often not achievable as some of our valuable drugs still have low therapeutic indexes eg. the opiates such as morphine and codeine.

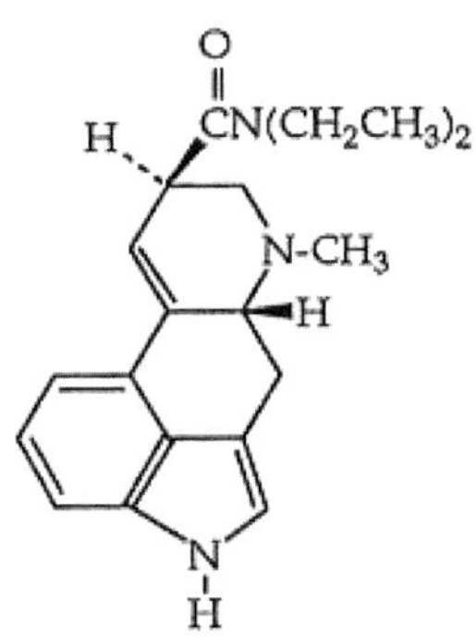


*Fig. 27. Structure of LSD*

LSD is usually taken by drug abusers as the tartrate salt in oral doses of 25-250 micrograms in the form of 'tickets' (absorbent paper containing the drug) quite often showing various logos:

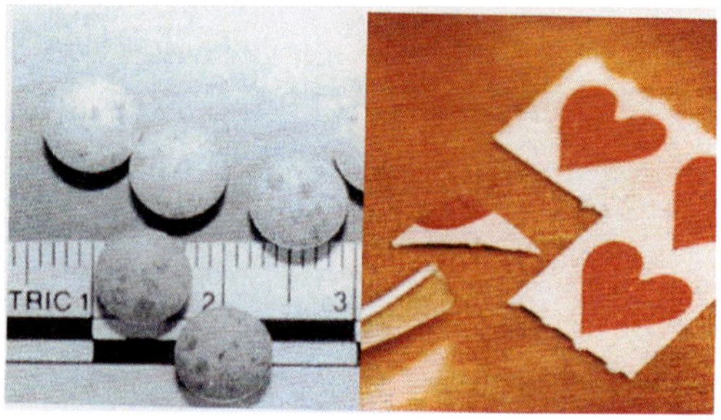


*Fig. 28. Some typical dosage forms of LSD*

Originally developed by Sandoz Laboratories, LSD was eventually abandoned as a clinical drug due to its unpredictable flashback side-effects and this made it very risky as a clinical drug. Yet amazingly it has still been used as a 'recreational' drug despite its unpredictable effects. However, some folk continued to use it from time to time when it was available, with unexpected results, as this case illustrates…

**The 'Problem'**

William ('Liam') Tully-Salter was considered 'a bit of a nuisance' by his so-called friends. He was part-aboriginal and believed friends should share everything. Everything – yes? His white 'friends' had different views. His taking of food and various other possessions was considered stealing and, not surprisingly, it was regarded as one of his shortcomings, and they were rapidly getting 'fed up' with his behaviour. However, in the aboriginal community this was a quality to be nurtured, as quite often this meant the survival of the community. Sadly, 'Liam' apparently did not seem to realise this in his new environment or chose to ignore it amongst his 'new friends' and the inappropriate group with whom he had aligned himself. To make things worse, they were regular drug users, which included the use of LSD – and large quantities of alcohol. This was to prove a fatal underestimation of the people he now associated with. He was now considered a 'problem' to be dealt with…

**Liam's Likeable Nature**

In actual fact Liam was an easy-going guy, and certainly did not deserve what later happened to him. One evening he was outside a Wollongong hotel and heard a band belting out a tune. 'Groovy man' was his reaction, and he sat on his backpack, put his surfboard on his knees and provided the beat. A young woman passing by heard his efforts and commented,

'He played on his surfboard like he was playing his bongos. It was really cool and he turned out to be a really good guy' and further, 'He hadn't been around long, he'd had some problems so he came to Wollongong to get away. He didn't even have a place to stay when we met him' and, 'Liam was just really friendly and nice.'

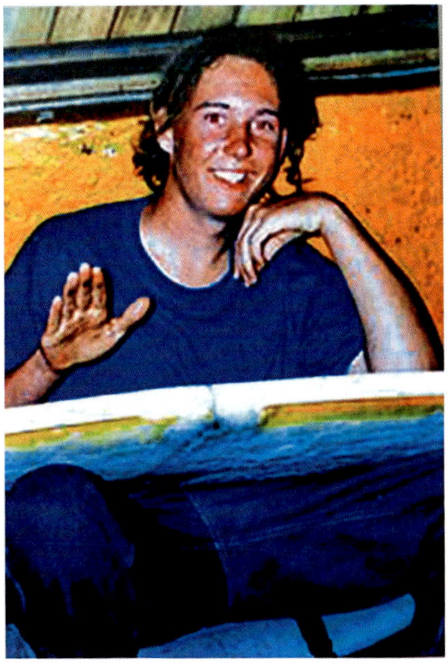

*Fig. 29. Liam Tully-Salter in happier days*
*[ Photo: AAP 2 May, 2002]*

**Plotting at the Pub**

Meanwhile, in the hotel a different point of view of Liam was expressed by Jason Farrell in particular, Daniel Ezold and Kai Purhonen. A lass by the name of Holly Turner was also present; her evidence was later to prove vital in this case. Little is known of the conversation which took place other than that it was to 'sort out the problem', but it became clear later that after consumption of an unknown quantity of alcohol and a 'ticket' of LSD or so by the participants, things were getting out of hand. Was there a pact? There was talk of a 'Musketeers-type threesome' with hands to carry out the evil deed. But who knows for certain? Whatever the situation, Liam's life was now in considerable danger.

A plan had emerged to 'sort out the problem'…

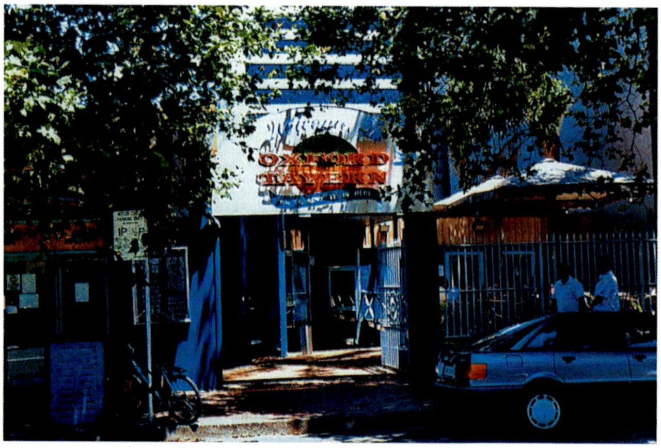

*Fig. 30. The Oxford Tavern, Wollongong – front view*

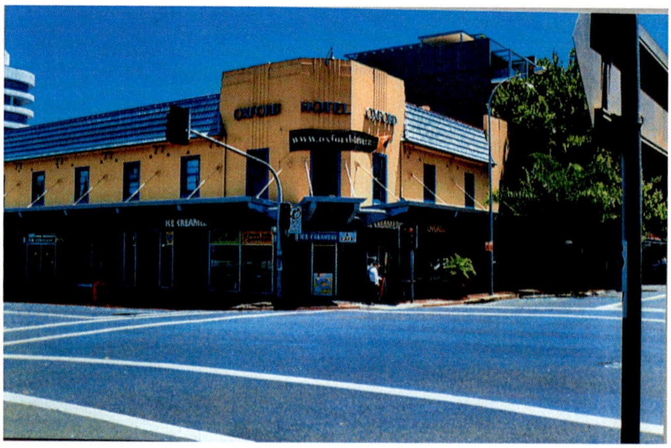

*Fig. 31. The Oxford Tavern, Wollongong – side view - where the plan emerged to 'sort out the problem'*
*Photos: Author*

### The Final 'Solution'

All parties eventually left the pub in various states of intoxication. Liam attended the group as they went for a walk to the Tom Thumb Lagoon in Wollongong. Previously, Ezold had worked in the area as a bush regenerator, and allegedly commented, "This would be a good place to get rid of someone." Then, without warning Ezold allegedly struck Liam with a 'Passion Pop' bottle, then Farrell grabbed the bottle off Ezold and continued with the bashing. He then kicked Liam down an embankment into a stormwater drain in the Tom Thumb Lagoon, near the grain terminal. The rest was now pure evil.

Liam was now held under the water with Farrell saying, "This is how Melbourne boys do it," and for some unknown reason said, "What is your mother's maiden name?"

Liam apparently just gurgled and was unable to say anything. Farrell called out to Daniel Ezold and Kai Purhonen to come and help him, they then both supposedly went to help him carry out the foul deed. Liam was repeatedly kicked before Farrell pushed his head under the muddy water for the final time, holding him there until there was no more movement. Liam's body was left in the culvert and the group walked to Wollongong beach. Farrell allegedly said to the trio that they should clean their clothing and footwear in the sea to wash away any evidence of the crime – and "I'm gonna celebrate with some scotch and a White Owl cigar tomorrow", "and I'll 'top off' anyone who talks" "I've done a few drownings."

His meaning and intention was quite clear to the group….

**'This is So Wrong'**

For two days after the death of Liam Saltwater, Holly sat on her couch in her flat oscillating between fear and guilt – sometimes both. Finally, she could not handle it any longer and decided to tell the Police because she said:

"There is a young man's body lying in a sewerage drain and it needs attention."

So she contacted Wollongong Police who, with the aid of the Rescue Squad, promptly found the deceased lying partly submerged in the dirty water. A crime scene was quickly established and detectives, including specialists, were called in to investigate.

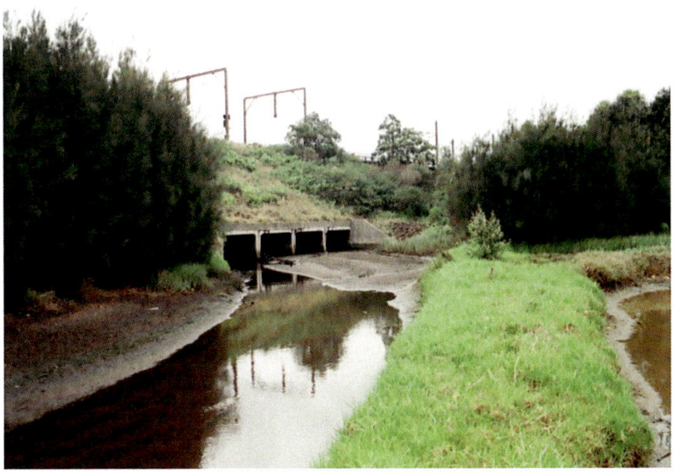

*Fig. 32. The culvert complex at Tom Thumb Lagoon*
*Photo: Wollongong Crime Scene, NSW Police Force.*

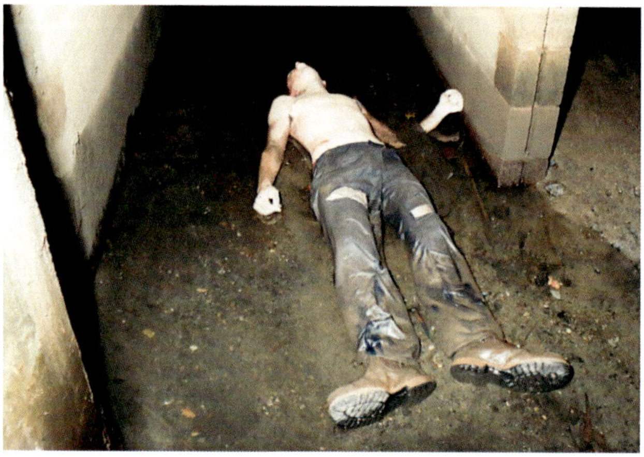

*Fig. 33. Liam's body in the culvert*
*Photo: Wollongong Crime Scene, NSW Police Force.*

**Physical Evidence**

Detective Greg Moon from the Wollongong Crime Scene Unit attended and described the crime scene in the following manner:

"At seven thirty p.m. on Saturday 18 November, 2000, I attended a command post located near the intersection of Springhill Road and Tom Thumb Road, Coniston. On my arrival I had a conversation with Senior Constable Maciver from the Police Rescue Squad. I was then shown the body of a male person who had been discovered underneath a stormwater tunnel there.

"The Tom Thumb Wetlands are located on the southern side of Springhill Road and on the northern side of a railway line accessing the coal and grain terminal at Port Kembla. The area comprises a tidal creek with medium-density vegetation. Included within this vegetation was a large quantity of 'Cobblers Peg' plants. There was a stormwater tunnel located underneath the railway line comprising of four separate tunnels. There was a steep embankment leading from the base of the stormwater tunnel, to the railway line above. These wetlands were tidal and attached to Port Kembla Inner Harbour. There was a bike track located between this vegetation and Springhill Road. The area of the stormwater tunnel was not visible from the road.

"The deceased was located in the last tunnel on the western side. He was found in a supine position with his head positioned towards the south. He was dressed in blue, work-type trousers; maroon underpants; brown work boots and brown socks.

"There was a T-shirt found on the western side of the deceased, partially wrapped around his left arm. Both legs were outstretched with the feet pointing outwards. His right arm was parallel with the torso. There were small abrasions around the knuckles of his right hand. The left arm was bent at the elbow and was positioned slightly away from the body. His left hand was resting against the support wall in the centre of the tunnel. There were abrasions to his left hand.

There was also a small abrasion on the right side of his stomach. Partial rigor mortis was still present in the body.

"There was mould located around the head of the deceased and on both sides of the stomach region. The entire body was covered with dirt/silt, indicating that the deceased, at some time, had been totally immersed in water. The dirt/silt on top of his chest had dried. An orange-coloured tool [ a pair of secatures] was found in his back right pocket.

"Located on the western side of the tunnel between the deceased and the northern end of the tunnel were numerous shoe prints in the sand/mud. There was one full set of shoe prints which led right up to the deceased and back out again. The shoe prints closest to the body near the northern end of the support wall were just visible as they had been nearly washed away by tidal waters. The finer details were not visible and it appears that the water has run harder over these prints causing damage to the tread pattern. The remaining shoe prints nearer the exit tunnel were clearer with the tread pattern distinguishable. There were two further partial marks, which appeared to be a different shoe print. One of these prints was located underneath the other shoe prints, indicating that this print was left prior to the others. Later, I [Detective Moon] made three plaster cast moulds of these shoe prints.

"I conducted a presumptive test for blood where the body had been located, using the chemical Luminol. Luminol is a chemical used to locate bloodstains that are difficult to see or invisible to the naked eye. When Luminol and blood react together, a chemical reaction takes place and blue light is produced. The area above the north western corner of the stormwater tunnel luminesced. The luminescence stopped approximately one metre along the western edge and two metres along the northern edge of the tunnel structure. This luminescence was visible for an area approximately one metre from the edge.

"Seen in the water approximately one metre from the northern end of the tunnel was a green bottle. The bottle was collected on Monday 20 November, 2000, after further information about the case was received."

During their usual search for clues, photographs were taken from various positions before Liam's body was pulled from the drain and conveyed to the Wollongong Morgue. Shortly afterwards the trio, Jason Farrell, Daniel James Ezold and Kai Purhonen were arrested and placed into custody.

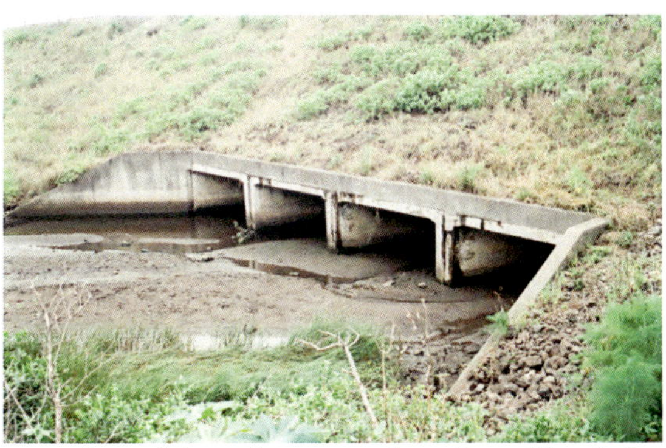

*Fig. 34. Close-up view of the culvert complex where Liam's body was found.*

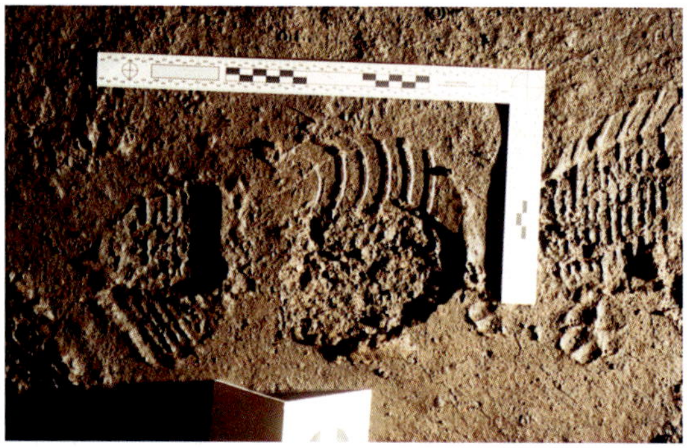

*Figs 35,36: Shoe prints near exit of culvert with distinguishable tread pattern.*

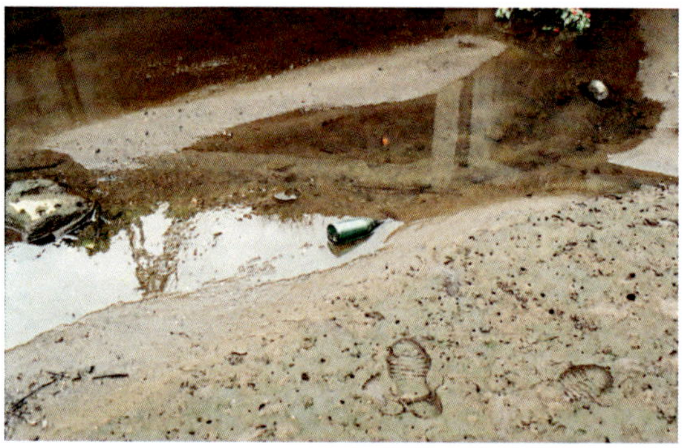

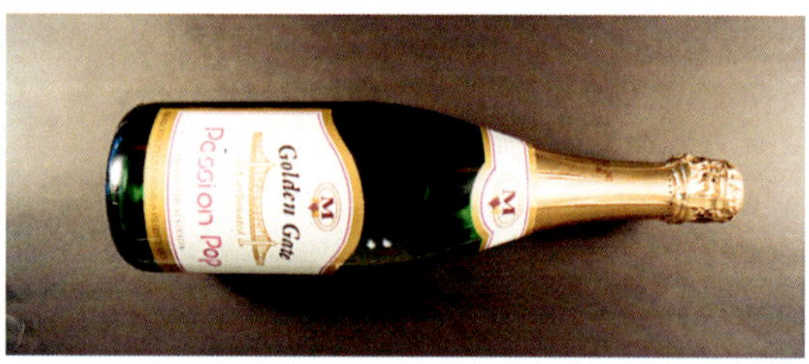


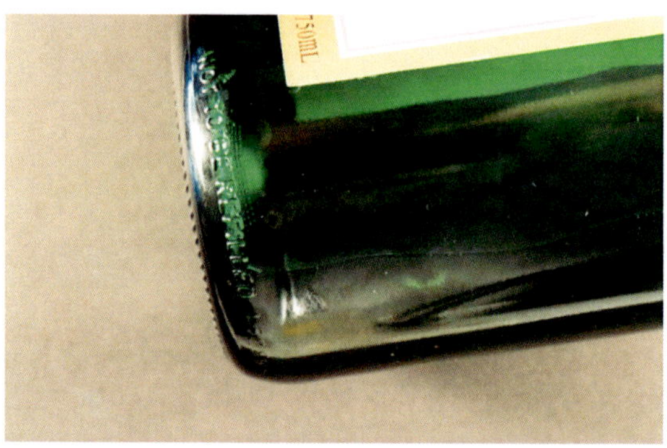

*Fig. 37a & b: Bottle used by Farrell.*
*Photos: Wollongong Crime Scene, NSW Police Force.*

**Search for Clues**

At three thirty a.m. on Sunday 19 November 2000, detectives attended Seaview Avenue, Coniston, armed with a search warrant, and later took possession of a large amount of clothing and footwear belonging to the three men in custody which the detectives soon took to their laboratory. The following afternoon, tests were carried out on these exhibits. During this time some dark red smears were found on the right sleeve of Jason Farrell's jacket (allegedly worn on the night of the murder) which tested positive for blood. Shortly afterwards his boots also gave a positive reaction. The same positive reaction occurred when they tested a pair of pants belonging to Daniel Ezold. Evidence was mounting against the pair but, unfortunately, none of the footwear seized by police matched any of the footprints found at the crime scene. However, it was later found that Holly's shoes did, in fact, match one of the patterns.

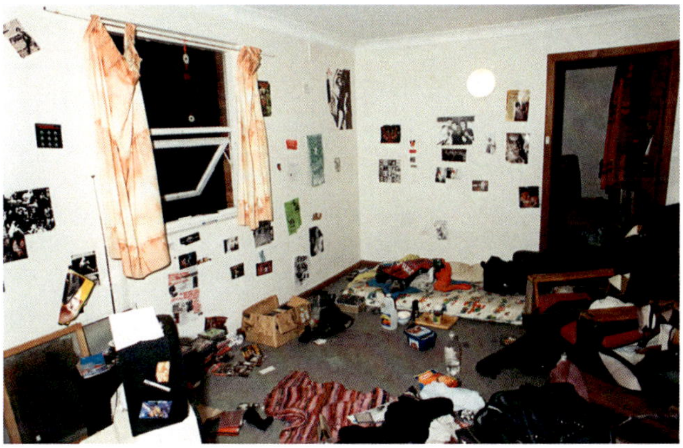

*Fig. 38*

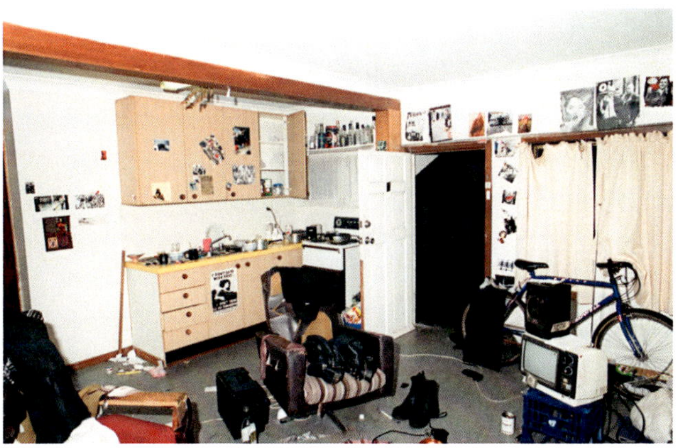

*Fig. 39*

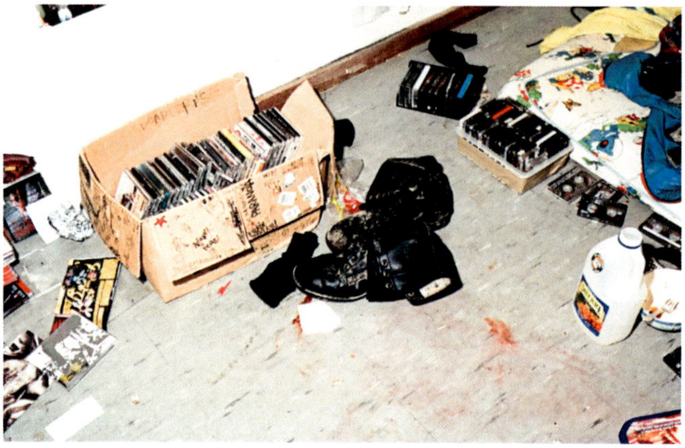

*Fig. 40.*

*Figs. 38, 39, 40: The scenes confronting police when they searched the Seaview Avenue premises.*

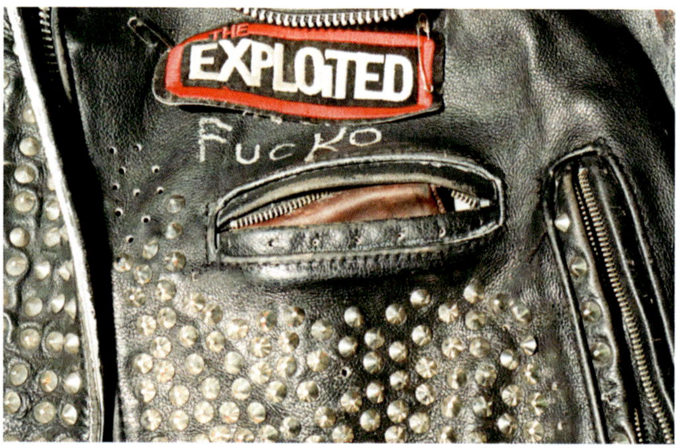


*Fig. 41.*

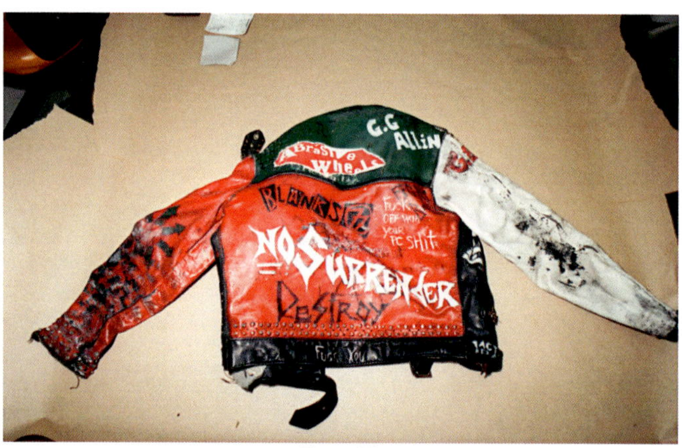


*Fig. 42.*

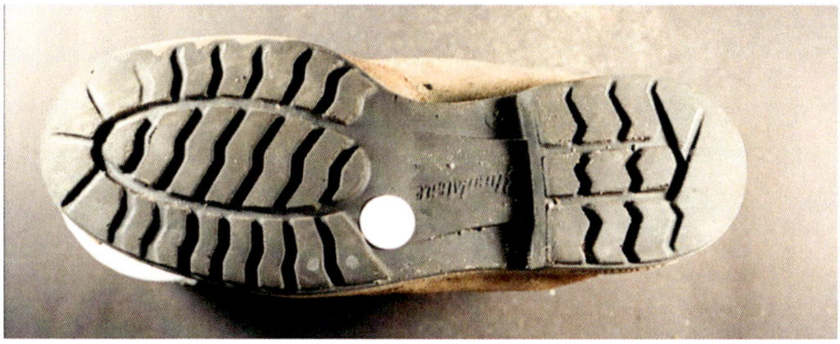

*Fig. 43.*

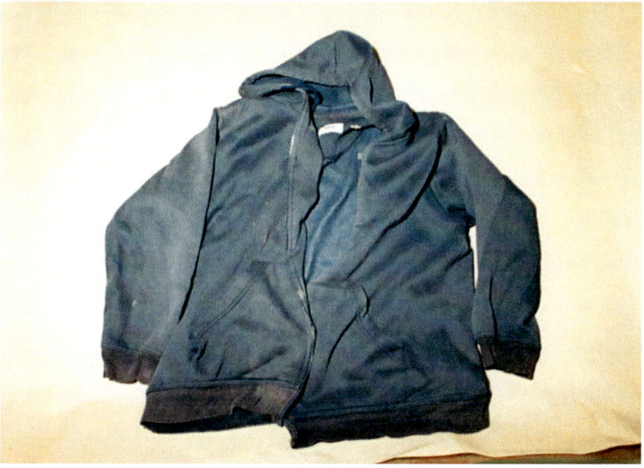

*Fig. 44.*

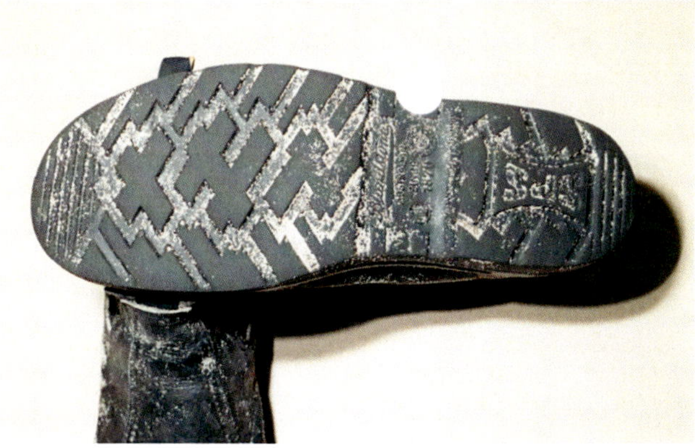

*Fig. 45.*

*Figs 41 - 45:Clothing and footwear taken by police for testing. [Photos: Wollongong Crime Scene, NSW Police Force.]*

## Post Mortem

Meanwhile, the necessary post-mortem examination was carried out at the Institute of Forensic Medicine, Glebe. The examination was conducted by Dr Cala and his assistant Dr Sugo. Later Dr Cala reported (in part): "The cadaver showed evidence of mould on the arms and flanks and moderated decomposition change to the face, neck and upper chest region. It is alleged that the deceased may have been thieving property and other items from those whom he had been associating. It is alleged that the deceased was assaulted above a large stormwater drain or similar water conveying channel before then possibly pushed down into the stormwater drain and forcibly held under the water which was present in the drain at the time. The exact time that he was held under the water is unclear, however there is a suggestion it may have been long as five to ten minutes. The lungs appeared hyper expanded, however, there was no obvious fluid within the airways. These findings are very suggestive, if not diagnostic for, drowning.

"Internal examination showed the presence of gravel or similar material in the upper and lower airways extending to the periphery of both lungs and is indicative the deceased was alive at the time he was allegedly pushed into the stormwater drain."

The post mortem of Liam's body revealed that he had indeed fought for his life in the final minutes before his death. There was evidence that the teenager had struggled desperately to breathe minutes before he drowned in the stormwater culvert. Sand particles and grit were found deep in Liam's windpipe revealed the extent of his struggle for life. It would have been a very terrifying and cruel end for a young man barely seventeen years of age. At the completion of the post mortem, Detective Moon took possession of the following exhibits and specimens found on the deceased: (i) empty packet of Gitanes cigarettes and a green cigarette lighter collected from the victim's pants; (ii) pair of secatures; (iii) pair of work boots; (iv) pair of socks; (v) blue work trousers; (vi) maroon underpants; (vii) 'Quicksilver' T-shirt; (viii) blood for grouping; (ix) an oropharangeal swab; (x) recal swab; (xi) left fingernails; (xii) right fingernails; (xiii) head hair; (xiv) pubic hair and (xv) sand/grit collected from the deceased's lungs.

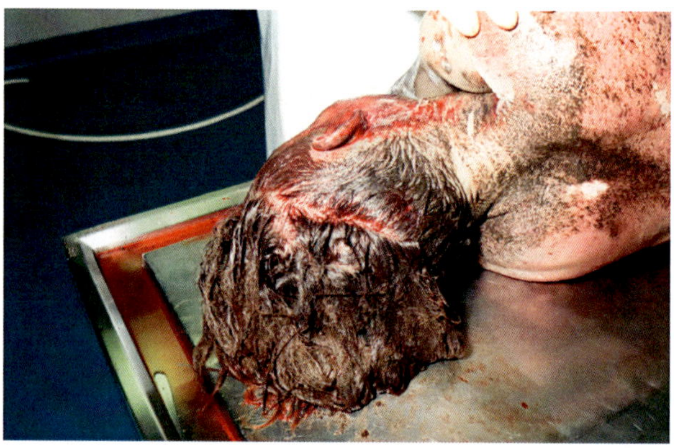

Fig. 46.

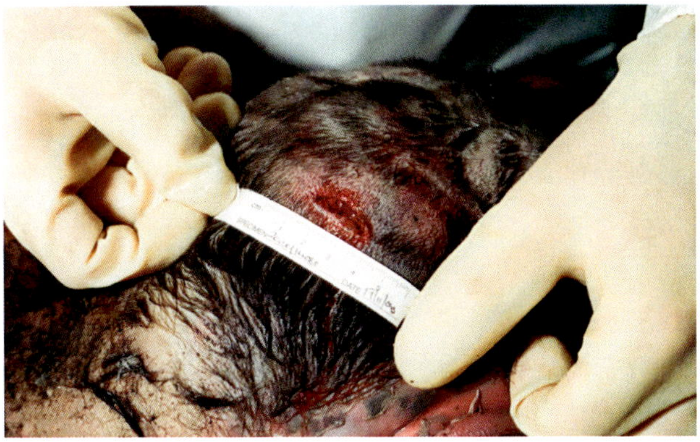

Fig. 47.

*Figs. 46, 47: Head injuries sustained by Liam*

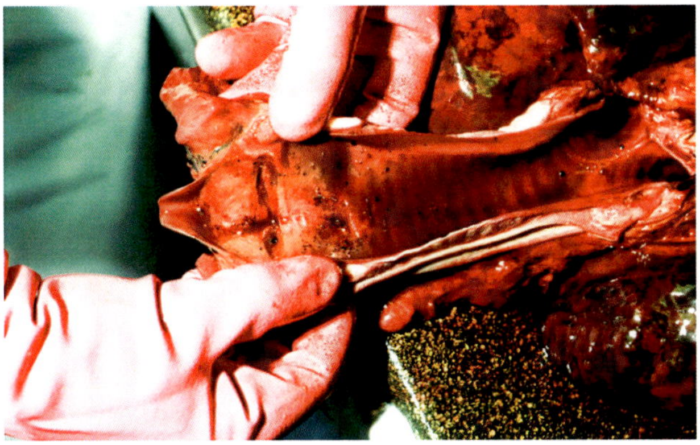

*Fig. 48: Grit and sand found in Liam's trachea (windpipe).*
*[Photos: Wollongong Crime Scene, NSW Police Force.]*

## Trials and Tribulations

The three nineteen-year-olds Jason Farrell, Daniel Ezold and Kai Purhonen, all of Seaview Road, Coniston, Wollongong were soon charged with Liam's murder.

The matter subsequently went before the courts where evidence was given that Jason Farrell seemed "excited" over the prospect of having bashed and drowned Liam Tully-Salter at the Tom Thumb Lagoon. Evidence was given that shortly after the murder Farrell was allegedly: "high, singing and skipping and making jokes about it." Moreover, the jury was told how Farrell struck Liam on the head with a bottle and then kicked him down an embankment into a stormwater drain. The victim was then held under the water until "his face was blue" as he died.

Farrell pleaded not guilty to murder, but guilty to manslaughter on the grounds he was very intoxicated at the time. The jury heard earlier that he was "off his face" with a combination of alcohol and LSD.

The NSW Supreme Court then heard that the next co-accused, Daniel Ezold, drank daily to excess and was well on his way to becoming an alcoholic. In addition, he was a regular drug user. On the night Liam was bashed and drowned, Ezold had taken a "trip and a half of LSD" and had consumed a large quantity of wine. Liam Tully-Salter was also on drugs and had been drinking heavily on the night he was murdered. (LSD was detected in a urine sample taken from Liam's body at post-mortem confirming he had also taken the drug.) Therefore, Liam's ability to defend himself would have been compromised through a combination of alcohol and LSD. However, for some unknown reason the level of alcohol in his blood was never fully ascertained.

The suggestion of an agreement between Daniel Ezold, Jason Farrell and Kai Purhonen was raised in carrying out the assault and subsequent murder of Liam, of Liam Tully-Salter. When asked about this, Ezold said, "We were friends, [and ironically] lifers, we were friends for life." Later he added, *"It was just a bit of drunken nonsense."*

The defence barrister, Mr Gordon said the Crown had no reliable evidence that there had been a pact to harm Liam Tully-Salter. Ezold said he did not recall anything about the death of Liam Tully-Salter and was supposedly shocked to have heard the allegations. "I'm blown away. I don't expect to hear I've been out killing people."

**Unexpected Letter**

However, two weeks later he wrote a letter in gaol, detailing his alleged involvement in the murder – a letter of remorse and guilt, in which, in part, he wrote: "We walked down to Tom Thumb Lagoon, because I thought it would be a good place to get rid of someone. I hit Liam over the head with a Passion Pop bottle and kicked him a couple of times." He then indicated that Farrell (who was apparently the ringleader of the group), allegedly grabbed the bottle off Ezold and continued with the bashing until he was unconscious. "Don't hate me," he continued, "It's not a hard step to kill. I might get off with manslaughter. I didn't actually kill him, just helped with the process."

Detectives, of course, had already noted that on the night in question, Ezold had taken a 'trip and a half' of LSD and was allegedly drinking from a second cask of wine. So, given the amount of alcohol he apparently consumed, it is difficult to discern how he was able to help "with the process" (of murder) except he must have developed a considerable tolerance to alcohol.

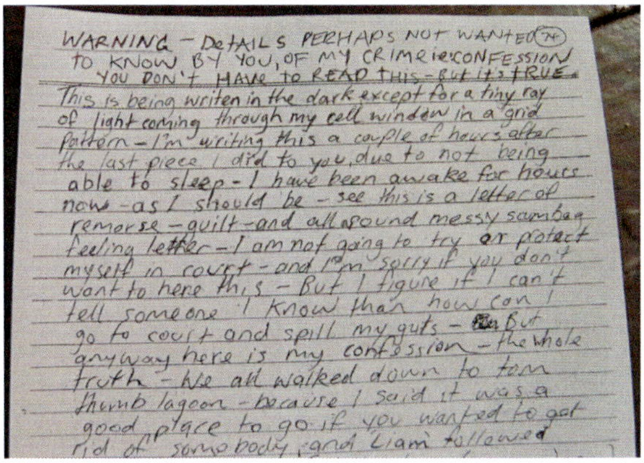

WARNING – DETAILS PERHAPS NOT WANTED TO KNOW BY YOU, OF MY CRIME ie:CONFESSION
YOU DON'T HAVE TO READ THIS – But it's TRUE.
This is being writen in the dark except for a tiny ray of light coming through my cell window in a grid pattern – I'm writing this a couple of hours after the last piece I did to you, due to not being able to sleep – I have been awake for hours now – as I should be – see this is a letter of remorse – guilt – and all round messy sambag feeling letter – I am not going to try or protect myself in court – and I'm sorry if you don't want to here this – But I figure if I can't tell someone I know than how can I go to court and spill my guts – But anyway here is my confession – the whole truth – We all walked down to tom thumb lagoon – because I said it was a good place to go if you wanted to get rid of somebody, and Liam followed

*Figs 49 a & b: Part of the letter written by Daniel Ezold whilst in gaol.*

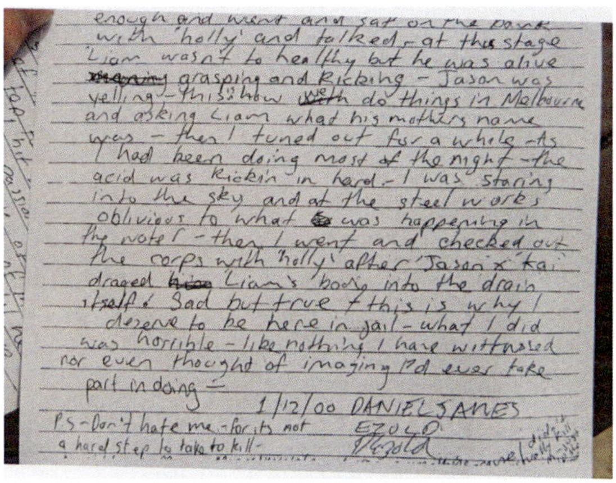

enough and went and sat on the bank with 'holly' and talked – at this stage Liam wasn't to healthy but he was alive grasping and kicking – Jason was yelling – this is how with do things in Melbourne and asking Liam what his mothers name was – then I tuned out for a while – As I had been doing most of the night – the acid was kickin in hard – I was staring into the sky and at the steel works oblivious to what was happening in the water – then I went and checked out the corps with 'holly' after Jason & Kai draged Liam's body into the drain itself. Sad but true & this is why I deserve to be here in jail – what I did was horrible – like nothing I have wittnesed nor even thought of imaging I'd ever take part in doing –

1/12/00 DANIEL JAMES EZOLD

PS – Don't hate me – for it's not a hard step to take to kill –

D Ezold

**Last But Not Least**

The third co-accused, Kai Purhonen, a Wollongong punk rocker, appeared to be in a more complex situation. He was charged as a accessory to murder, but was not committed to trial, and at the time not required to enter a plea. This became somewhat doubtful as to how much he was involved in the assault, which led to Liam's death. Purhonen appeared to have stood by and watch Tully-Salter die.

"This defendant [Purhonen] stood by and watched him die."

This didn't seem to indicate active involvement, whilst other evidence seemed to indicate he did.

The defence council stated: "Clearly, he was not at the forefront of this unhappy crime" and he appeared to have been affected by LSD and alcohol at the time of the murder. Nevertheless, Kai Purhonen, a bass player with the band Blurred Vision, would spend almost eighteen months in custody waiting to prove his innocence. In the meantime, Farrell would be gaoled for eighteen years and Ezold for sixteen years.

## Court

The appalling murder had been committed on the evening of 15 November, 2000. But it wasn't until 2004 when I, along with Professor Graham Starmer of Sydney University, were subpoenaed to appear in the Supreme Court. Therefore the matter had been running on and off for close to four years!

I appeared in Supreme Court in Sydney on 3 May, 2004 and gave evidence as to the effects of LSD on a person's faculties and sensibilities. This was not an easy call, as I did not know whether Purhonen was a regular user or not. However, the "wavy lines" brought up in evidence did seem to indicate some affectation by a drug, but could also be from other mental problems on which I was not qualified to comment. After a three-week hearing, the jury took just half an hour to clear Kai Purhonen of murder. They rejected evidence from a female witness (Holly) that he was involved, and accepted his version that he did not know what was happening until it was too late. Given the alleged quantity of alcohol consumed, along with the LSD, I had to agree with them!

## A Troubled Young Man

Ordinarily, he should have been allowed to go free on the day he was acquitted.

Unfortunately, it took another month to secure him Supreme Court bail, due to several other charges including an incident at the Oxford Tavern where he defended himself against taunts and jeers. He was charged with wounding and his bail was revoked. He then waited the next five months in custody before his murder trial in the NSW Supreme Court. Eventually, these were finalised in a two-day hearing in Wollongong Court. Gaol had left him withdrawn and depressed. His creativity was apparently sapped by his experiences, and he no longer played music. Instead he fought depression and drank heavily to lessen the pain. His best friend, Corinne Smith said, "He'd seen a lot of things in gaol but he'd never tell me about them." Nonetheless this period had a profound effect on his outlook on life, which was hardly surprising.

## Final Outcome

For Kai Purhonen the toll of the last four years had become too much and he committed suicide by hanging. When he took his own life, he was still 'living in his own private gaol' and to those who knew him this was no surprise, although his method of departure was. Naturally, his family were very angry that even his acquittal did not end his ordeal. They felt that he should have been released from prison with some form of back-up, which included counselling, medication and support services, which were apparently not forthcoming. Unfortunately, this scenario is fairly common for released prisoners, which may account for re-offenders!

Kai Purhonen summed up his own position thus:“I don’t know how this thing has happened. If only everyone could look into my eyes and see that I didn’t kill this man. I’m dying to live.”

## Conclusion

He went to his grave without any criminal convictions, and guests were urged to bring a tree to plant in his honour. In summation, police had to deal with two pointless deaths of young persons resulting from “just a bit of drunken nonsense” – and a tragic corpse in a culvert…

# 6
# No Laughing Matter

*"I used to always think that I'd look back on us crying and laugh, but, I never thought I'd look back on us laughing and cry."*

Ralph Waldo Emerson

## Introduction

This case involved the use of nitrous oxide – known a 'laughing gas' – and a paedophile who was in a position of trust in the community. But firstly, a bit of background on the 'drug' used in the various offences. Nitrous oxide is a gaseous substance which has been used in dentistry and medicine for over 150 years. Joseph Priestly first discovered it in 1776, and although its potential as an anaesthetic was recognised by Humphrey Davy in 1799, it did not come into general usage until after 1860. The nonflammable, nearly odourless gas with a slight sweetish smell, is a good analgesic, but will not produce complete anaesthesia at safe concentrations (65% oxygen) and so is used mainly as an analgesic (pain relieving) agent in dentistry. Nitrous oxide is relatively insoluble in body tissues and fluids and so induction and recovery are generally quite rapid. Due to its effects before anaesthesia, nitrous oxide is also known as 'laughing gas' as it had the effect of producing a type of 'laugh' and so was used recreationally at parties, much like Ecstasy is used in rave parties today.

Inhalation of 40% nitrous oxide in air causes confusion and sedation, while a level of 80% causes unconsciousness in most people.

*Fig. 50: Structures of nitrous oxide*

Nitrous oxide is often inhaled recreationally for its euphoric effects, being readily obtained from whipped cream cans or from medical supplies. This gas is used as a propellant which mixes in the liquid cream. When the cream escapes from the can, the gas expands and in the process whips the cream into a foam. It is necessary to use a gas like nitrous oxide, as the more commonly used gas carbon dioxide would cause the cream to 'curdle' because of its acidic characteristics when dissolved in mixtures containing water.

This was a most curious case, where I was initially requested to comment on the use of nitrous oxide, which had allegedly been used in a number of sexual/ indecent assaults upon young male persons. The offence, paedophilia, whilst involving a person in a position of trust was, unfortunately, not unusual. Yet the means *used in the offence* did appear unusual…

**Church Youth Group**

It was midday on a warm Saturday in August 2000, when fifteen-year-old Scott Evers (not his real name) called around to 'Mr B's' ("Mr Buggers" – not his real name, but deemed appropriate at the time) residence at Dee Why, New South Wales. Previously, Scott had attended the youth group on a number of occasions on Friday night, where they played X-box, watched videos and played various other games. Yes, it was fun and in an apparently caring religious setting. He couldn't wait to meet his friends again. But today was going to be different – a different game using different tools… Scott knocked on the door, the curtains parted and Mr B, seeing his young charge, opened the door – another victim in the offering! Two of Scott's friends were already there, in various states of consciousness from nitrous oxide inhalation, and both had their shorts removed…

**The "Creaming Club"**

The person dubbed "Mr Buggers" was a youth leader at a Church group at Dee Why, Sydney. His position offered him the opportunity to indulge in his criminal conduct with teenage boys – and older. Apparently, the young boys and men were being sexually abused while under the influence of nitrous oxide, which had been inhaled through gas canisters attached to cream canisters for whipping liquid cream – minus the liquid cream.

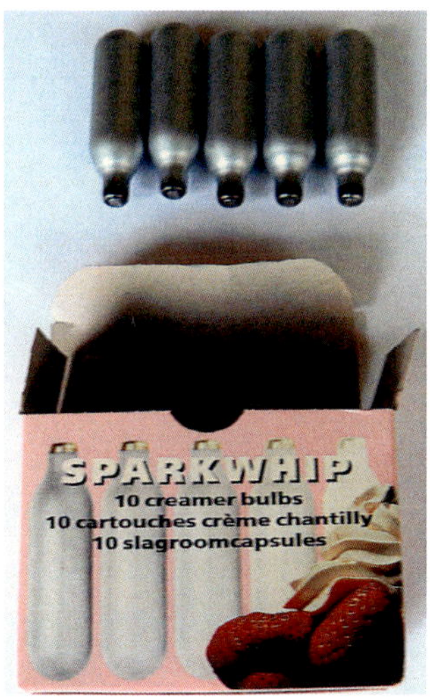


*Fig. 51: Typical bulbs of compressed nitrous oxide used to produce whipped cream.*

The victims were later asked by police, "So can you tell me what [Mr Buggers]'s has been up to? A victim replied, "Well he has this thing called a creaming club" [The bulb] "is put in, and screwed up" "Like the old-style creaming" … "you suck it in and then you get a high. And that's why he calls it the creaming club."

He was further asked, "And who else? Has anyone else ever done it before that you know of?" and he answered, "Yeah, a whole range of other people. He's got photos of them on his computer." ... "There's the creaming club and, and where does this, where do you go where the creaming club is, is it somewhere in..."

He further answered, "It's sometimes in his house and sometimes on the road."

This 'creaming club' was set up by Mr Buggers to incite young men ranging from eleven to twenty-three years to be sexual participants in his very deviate 'club'.

This club consisted of 'Mr Buggers' attracting various bored or otherwise unemployed male persons, to his 'lair' where he administered various doses of nitrous oxide to his 'prey'. This was via various creaming devices which were the nitrous oxide gas bulbs modified to deliver the gas to the victim.

Welcome to the 'creaming club'...

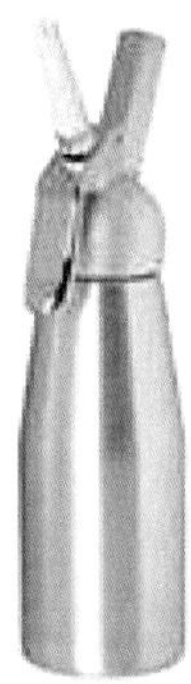

*Fig. 52: A similar creaming device found at "Mr Buggers" residence.*

**It's the Gas, but I'm not Laughing**

'Mr Buggers' provided the boys with canisters and bulbs of nitrous oxide and gave them instructions as to their use. The nitrous oxide was provided in such large quantities that the boys were rendered unconscious after a brief period of 'laughing' and various degrees of disinhibition, and were then sexually assaulted by 'Mr Buggers'. Eventually, one young 'member' could not stand it any more and reported Mr B's activities to the Police – who quickly acted accordingly, and nabbed the villain...

**Interviews by the police**

Police subsequently interviewed Mr B and his victims. It became quite evident from the initial interviews that Mr B had a pretty much a well worked out *modus operandi* using nitrous oxide capsules.

When asked by police, one of the victims replied, "he pulled out a little box of bulbs and he didn't put cream in to the actual whipper, he just put the bulbs into it and he showed me how to do it, then I passed out, 'cause it sometimes makes you pass out, and I woke up and he was feeling my private parts."

The victim was further asked, "When you, you woke up and he was first of all touching you and then he put his, his mouth over your penis, how were you feeling at the time?"

He answered, "I don't know."

"Do you have any recollection of what you felt like as a result of waking up after taking, using the stuff?"

He answered, "I still felt like I was stoned."

Further victims were interviewed regarding the activities of Mr B and the descriptions were disturbingly similar, with one, "Well, [Mr 'Buggers'], he pretty much, raped [another victim].

Mr B was subsequently charged with a number of offences relating to sexual/indecent assaults upon young male persons under Section 38 of the Crimes Act, that he 'did unlawfully cause to be taken chloroform or stupefying drug or thing to commit an indictable offence'.

This was followed by a request: "Doctor, can you say that nitrous oxide in your expert opinion is a stupefying drug or thing, and is disinhibiting or un-inhibiting to the user?'

Well, yes I could and did. As did other experts advised in the use of nitrous oxide; and these documents were submitted to Court in a rather large brief…

**Last 'laughs' – at Court**

This matter along with statements from various other experts and witnesses went before the District Court. The judge and jury were not amused. 'Mr B' was sentenced to thirteen years imprisonment with a non-parole period of nine and a half years. – Hopefully, by the time he is released he may have reflected on his former lifestyle and made appropriate amendments. But can a 'leopard change its spots'? Well, only time will tell…

# 7
# "Cuppa Anyone?"

*"To betray you must first belong."*

Harold Philby

## Introduction

Flunitrazepam is a drug which has featured frequently in various drug-facilitated sexual assaults (DFSAs) such that it became known as the 'date-rape drug'. Alarmed at the reputation the drug was getting, the drug company, Roche, changed the formulation to include a dye to warn of its presence in drinks and further, the Therapeutic Goods Administration (TGA) imposed further restrictions on the issue of drug. Along with other potent benzodiazepine relatives such as Mogadon (nitrazepam). This was a case which involved a drink spiking using another brand of flunitrazepam ('Hypnodorm') which unfortunately, at the time, did not contain a dye to warn of its presence in drinks.

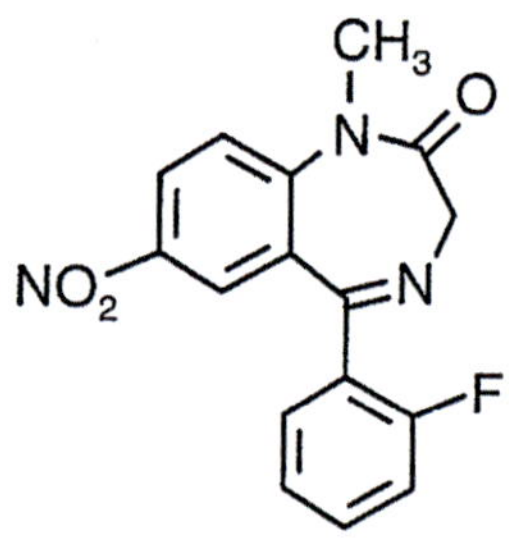


*Fig 53: Structure of flunitrazepam*

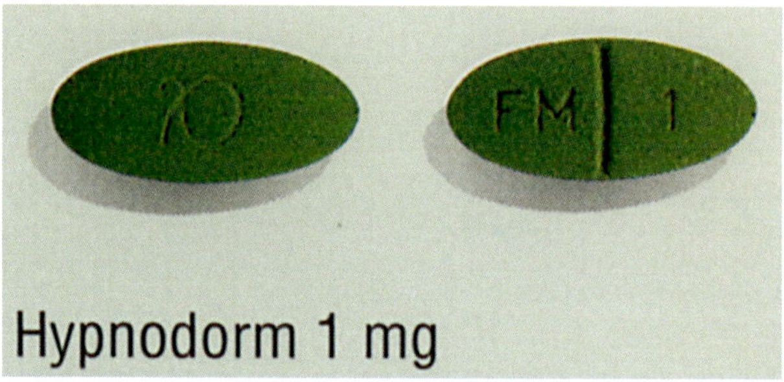


*Fig. 54: 'Hypnodorm' tablets*

Here the motive was to incapacitate the victims and rob them, one very wealthy…

## A 'Friendly' Fellow

It was a warm evening of 7 January, 2002 when Ian Campbell (not his real name) invited Saylit Bulut (alias 'Eric') to his humble residence, a granny flat, for a casual visit.

"Hi, Eric, good to see you again. Come join me here."

They sat outside the granny flat and engaged in animated conversation on various topics. 'Eric' later turns to 'Ian' and says, "Would you like a cuppa?"

"Yes, that would be nice," replies Ian.

'Eric' then goes into the flat and busies himself preparing their beverages, emerging some minutes later with two steaming mugs of tea. Ian consumes the tea commenting to 'Eric' that it was "somewhat bitter."

"I forgot to put in some sugar," replied Eric.

Ian consumed the remaining tea and after some minutes started to become drowsy and lethargic.

"Come on mate, I'll help you into the flat."

Eric then assisted Ian into his flat and laid him down onto a couch. By this time Ian was drifting in and out of semi-consciousness.

"I feel so sleepy…" he murmured, and drifted off into a deep sleep.

## Time for the Take

In the meantime 'Eric' was busy assessing anything of value in Ian's flat.

'Yep, it was a reasonable haul…' Some twelve hours later, Ian awakes from his deep sleep drowsy, and also nauseous. It was a rude awakening. He discovered that his so-called 'friend' had stolen property to the value of $40,000 from his flat. He then contacted police and reported the crime. Mr Campbell was taken to hospital where a sample of blood and urine were taken.

## Drug Levels Found

A blood sample taken from Mr Campbell at the St George Hospital at three thirty p.m. the following day was found to contain flunitrazepam at 0.006 milligrams per litre (mg/L). I found this level was quite significant given the long time interval, and suspected more than the therapeutic dosage had been given to the victim.

[Also detected was the drug, nevirapine. This latter drug indicated that the victim was being medicated for HIV-1.]

But, Mr Bulut was still busy, and just over a year later he struck again…

## 2 A Thai Collection

On the morning of eight twenty a.m. on 23 March 2003 Sayit Bulut visited a Thai transsexual (born a male, who had adopted the appearance of a female). With a similar *modus operandi,* he befriended the victim and offered 'Chris Nixon' (not his/her real name) a cup of coffee. A short time later 'Chris' slips into an unconsciousness state and after some seven a half hours later, awakes in a very drowsy state. In the meantime a large amount of property in the form of jewellery was stolen while Chris was in a deep state of sleep. Clearly, Mr Bulut could not believe his luck, this person was very wealthy and so he took advantage of the situation…

### Count the Cost

When Chris gained consciousness, it was discovered that the so-called casual 'friend' had stolen jewellery to the value of nearly *two million dollars*!!

Police were promptly contacted and the crime reported. Ms Nixon was taken to hospital where a sample of this person's blood and urine were taken.

### Drug Levels Found

A blood sample taken from Ms. Nixon at the hospital at five thirty p.m. that day was found to contain flunitrazepam at 0.006 milligrams per litre (mg/L). However, MDMA ( our old friend Ecstasy) was also detected in his/her urine. I found this level was quite significant given the long time interval, and suspected more than the therapeutic dosage had also been given to this victim. The presence of MDMA (3,4 – methylenedioxymethylamphetamine or Ecstasy) in his/her urine appeared to be puzzling at the time. Its presence may have accounted for the ease with which Bulut was able to befriend Ms Nixon – and administer the drug in his/her coffee.

MDMA whilst being a stimulant drug, also tends to make the consumer more sociable and friendly. Such that it has been called an entactogen or 'hug drug' and even the 'street name' Ecstasy gives a hint as to its popularity in a social and/or 'rave' scene. However, no MDMA was detected in his/her blood so it was difficult to determine whether this contributed to the victim's impairment!

### The Trial and Outcome

The matter went before the District Court in the presence of a jury. I was called to provide expert testimony in relation to the pharmacological effects of flunitrazepam found in the blood of both of the victims. I mentioned that flunitrazepam is a potent benzodiazepine-type drug that has central nervous system (CNS) depressant effects, and that it produces a sedative effect, amnesia, muscle relaxation and a slowing of psychomotor responses with a rapid onset of action occurring some twenty to thirty minutes after ingesting the drug. However, the effects of the drug are long lasting. Further questions included:

"Doctor, in regard to the particular charges before the Court, the allegation that the accused did administer a stupefying drug. Does this drug have the capacity to cause one to fall into a stupor?

I said, "Absolutely. With only a milligram dose, the blood levels of flunitrazepam would peak at about forty-five minutes after ingestion, and fall to one half after the peak after twenty to thirty hours."

One victim clearly had more than this. The amount of flunitrazepam detected after sixteen hours was consistent with the ingestion of greater than a therapeutic dose of flunitrazepam.

Mr Bulut was found guilty and sentenced to seven years imprisonment. Hopefully, by the time he is released he may have reflected on his former lifestyle and made appropriate amendments…

# 8
# The Westpac Bank Robbery "Steroids Made Me Do It!"

*"There are some things so serious you have to laugh at them."*

Niels Bohr

## Another day, another dollar

It was a warm Saturday morning of 20 December 2003, when Susan Aquino the branch manageress of Westpac Bank at Auburn, Sydney arrived at the bank just before eight thirty a.m. On her arrival, staff rostered to work at the bank that day, were at the front entrance waiting to be let in. Also waiting was an electrician to fix an air conditioner. Ms Aquino entered the bank and carried out various safety checks, alarms and locks. On satisfactory completion, the awaiting staff members entered the bank to commence business. But unfortunately, this was not going to be an ordinary working day…

As staff started to walk in to the bank, they were followed by what appeared to be two 'Telstra' workers. They were dressed as 'Telstra' workers but, curiously, they had workers' hats, dark glasses – and white dust masks over their faces! One spoke to Ms Aquino and said:

"We're going to do some work for Telstra and electricity," which he repeated. Ms Aquino was suspicious as they showed no personal identification. But it was too late; the robbers had gained entrance to the bank, followed by a third bandit. After successfully gaining entry to the bank, their true motives were revealed…

## The Robbery

The staff was then told by one of the tall robbers,

"All of youse come in here, and lie face down on the floor, and stop looking at us."

The tallest bandit had a white dust mask on his face, a straw-style hat on his head, he was wearing an orange safety vest and black sunglasses. This bandit was later identified as Jamil Jaafar. His two shorter accomplices wore white hardhats and also had an orange safety vest.

He demanded, "We want the ATM money. Who's in charge here?

Ms Aquino said, "It's me."

"Then open the ATM," he growled.

"I cannot because I don't have the combination," she said.

"Why is that?" the shorter robber said, waving a Taser menacingly in his hand.

"The girl who does it is not here today. We don't open them on the weekend," she replied nervously, reaching for the silent alarm button under the desk.

"All right then, we want the treasury money," the tall robber said, as he produced a Luger pistol from his trousers.

Anger and confusion then rippled through Susan Aquino as she looked into the face of the brawny young man wearing an orange safety vest and black sunglasses. His outfit was farcical, but he was pointing a Luger at her.

"I'll take you to the main bank safe," she said, glancing at the weapon, and took the two robbers to the bank safe.

In the meantime, the third robber tied up the other bank staff using cable ties.

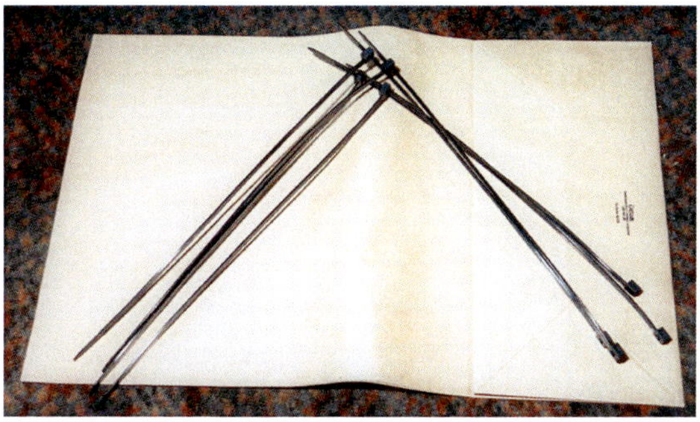

*Fig. 55: The cable ties used to tie up the bank employees during the robbery. [Photo: Bass Hill Crime Scene, NSW Police Force]*

Eventually, after some difficulties, Susan obtained the codes for the main safe which allowed access to the main money supply ('the treasury') held by the bank. As the main safe had a time delay, there was some tension with one robber saying, "Are you delaying?" as they took the tellers' money from the other safes.

Ms Aquino replying, "No, the keys wouldn't fit in."

One calm and brave lady, who had a weapon pointed at her during most of the robbery.

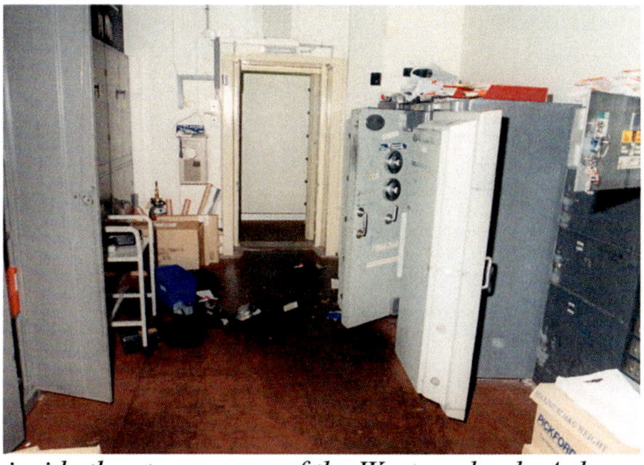

*Fig. 56: View inside the strongroom of the Westpac bank, Auburn Road, Auburn [Photo: Bass Hill Crime Scene, NSW Police Force]*

**A Bag Full of Dollars**

In the intervening time the treasury safe opened, and Susan opened the door and the tall robber, Jaafar, reached in and took a container of money and emptied it into the black bag, along with a number of foreign currencies.

[Later, the haul proved to be very impressive, which consisted of $68,559.60 Australian dollars, $43,824 USA dollars, $1300 Euros, $320 Franks and $300 Fiji dollars.]

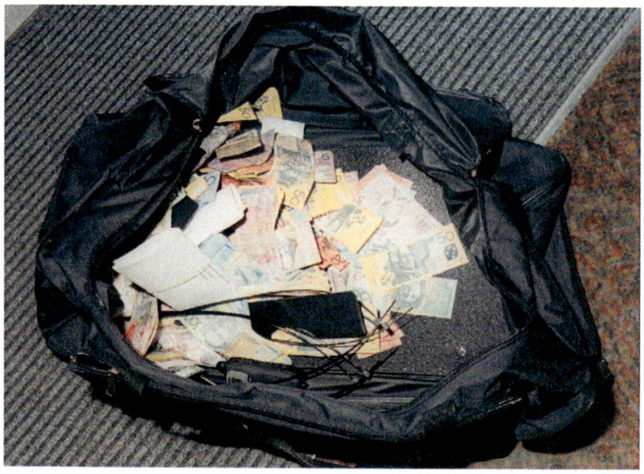

*Fig. 57: View of the contents inside the large black bag*

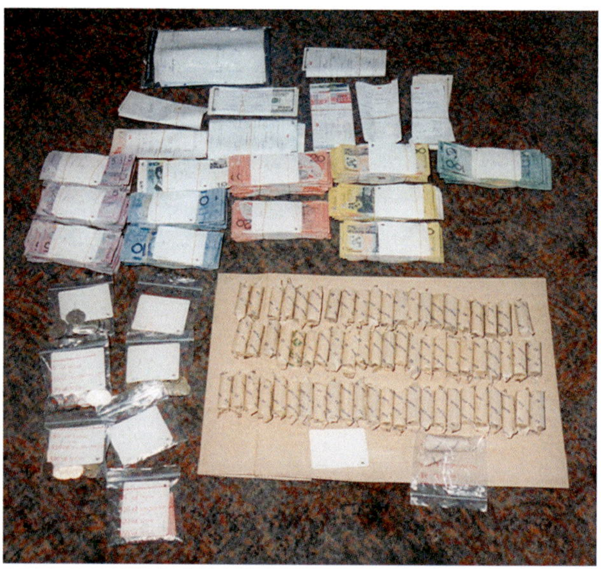

*Fig. 58: View of the money and bank documents removed from inside the large black bag.*

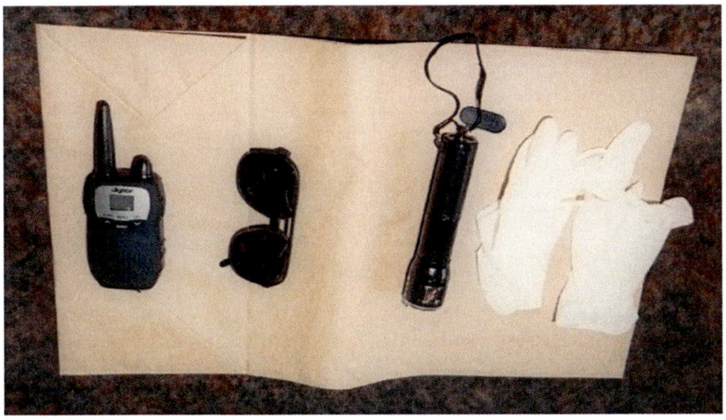

*Fig. 59: View of a 'Digitor' scanner, sunglasses, torch and disposable gloves also removed from inside the large black bag.*
*[Photos: Bass Hill Crime Scene, NSW Police Force]*

Suddenly, the walkie-talkie crackled into life with voice of the third accomplice, "The cops are outside."

The short robber said, "Hurry up, open the door."

The manageress walked to the front door of the bank and, seeing no one was there, pressed the button and the doors opened. All of the robbers ran through the door into the arms of the police! Police who had, in the meantime, been contacted and were waiting for them…

[The black bag containing its valuable contents, was dropped on the floor at the bank's entrance!!]

**Drop the gun!**

Unfortunately for the police, all three of the robbers made their alternative means of escape. The tall robber Jamil Jaafar chose, somewhat unwisely, to rely on a firearm in his pocket. He started to walk towards the ANZ bank and placed his right hand on the handle of the firearm. He then removed the firearm (a 9mm Luger pistol) from his strides and raised it towards the police. Detective Senior Constable Paul Arnold (Auburn Detectives) drew his pistol and, recognising the potential danger to himself and the other police present, yelled out to Jamil Jaafar, "Put the fucking gun down, put the fucking gun down!"

At the time there were a number of other police officers present who also had their firearms drawn and pointed at Jaafar. There were further repeated directions from the police for him to put the firearm down. Eventually, he realised he was outnumbered and, after some further hesitation, eventually placed the weapon into a nearby garbage bin.

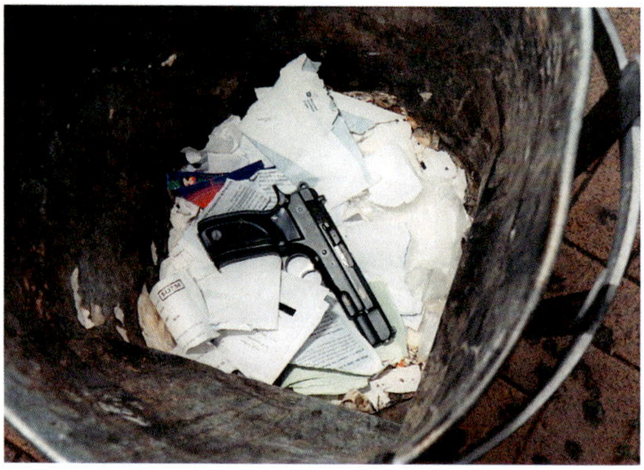

*Fig. 60:View of the 9mm "Lugar" handgun inside the council bin at Auburn, NSW*

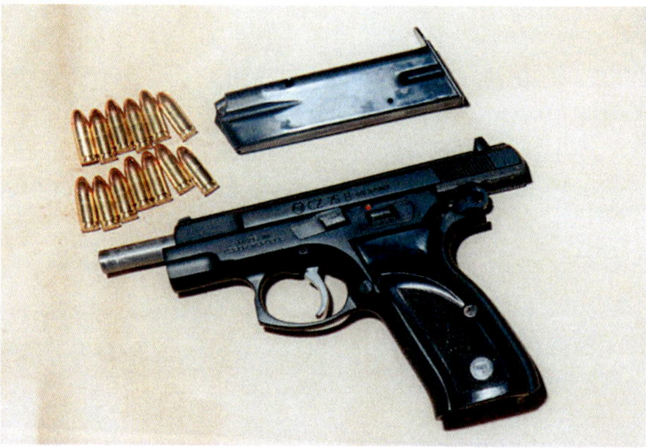

*Fig. 61: View of the 9mm "Lugar" handgun with the magazine removed and thirteen (13) live 9mm bullets also removed from the magazine.*
*[Photos: Bass Hill Crime Scene, NSW Police Force]*

He was subsequently wrestled to the ground by police officers, sprayed with oleoresin capsicum (OC) spray and handcuffed.

The handgun Jaafar had in his possession was a 9 mm 'Parabellum' calibre CZ manufactured self-loading pistol. The serial number had been removed, and there were thirteen live rounds in the magazine, of a maximum of fifteen. – And clearly, he meant business…

**Getaways**

As the Police were dealing with Jaafar, accomplice two was seen to get into a blue Subaru WRX motor vehicle and after accelerating harshly, drove south along Auburn Road. As this happened, a number of police officers had to get out of the way to avoid being hit by the vehicle.

Accomplice three chose another means of escaping, which was tracked to the rear of Coles supermarket where police were unable to find him after a good deal of searching.

A number of items had been discarded including a "Uniden" handheld scanner, in his quest to avoid capture.

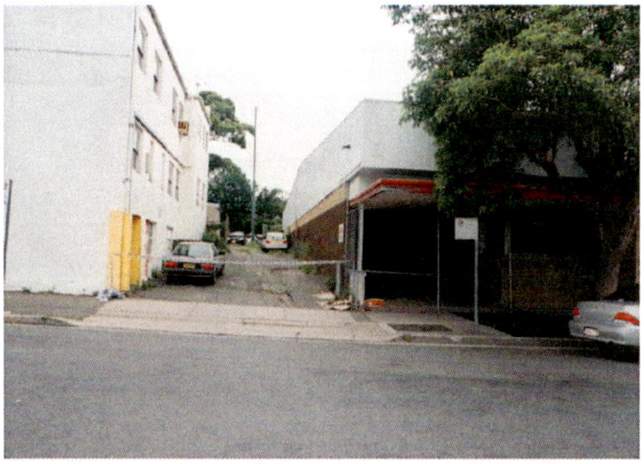

*Fig. 62: General easterly view from Mary Street, Auburn looking towards the small lane way.*

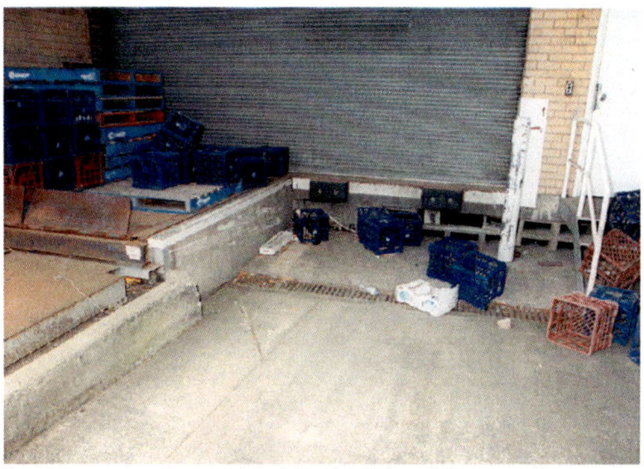

*Fig. 63: View of dock area of an old 'Coles' building where the third accomplice apparently escaped.*

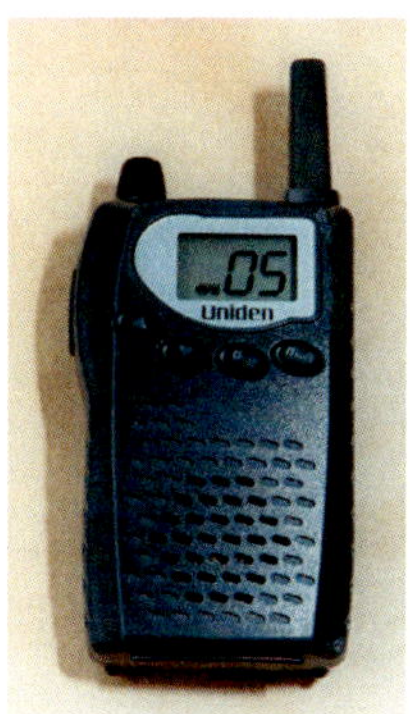


*Fig. 64: Close view of the front of a "Uniden" handheld scanner discarded in the dock area at the rear of the old Coles building in Harrow Road, Auburn. [Photos: Bass Hill Crime Scene, NSW Police Force]*

Jaafar was taken to Auburn Police station where he was electronically interviewed. He was later charged with a number of offences including: robbery, armed with an offensive weapon.

**The Initial Court proceedings**

On June 21 2004, Jamil Jaafar was committed at Burwood Court house where bail was refused, and the matter was then committed to the District Court at Sydney on July 2, 2004. Meanwhile, Mr Jaafar sought a novel defence for his actions and, through a solicitor, obtained the services of a consultant psychologist and criminologist: Mr Peter Clark-Saunders…

**Steroids – and more Steroids**

It seems Mr Jaafar was keen to improve his body image as he was 'extremely overweight as a child' and so took to the gym. However, to speed up his physical development, he supposedly embarked on a course of steroids between the age of seventeen and eighteen years old to achieve this aim. He was apparently, ninetten years old at the time of the offence. A variety of anabolic and androgenic steroids have been used (and abused) in gyms to bolster muscle mass. No doubt this continues to be the situation. However, this was used as a defence for his actions and probably also to reduce his sentence, which then became "steroid-induced rage".

That is, "his judgement was affected at the time [of the offence] by his steroid use" or that "steroids made me [Jaafar] do it." "I was high on steroids and I was out of control." This is appears to be where the problem began – and to the crime.

Mr Jaafar began injecting the following anabolic steroids namely, Sustanon (one of several trade names for testosterone); Stanazole (a trade name for stanozol) and Decka 50 or Deca durabolin (a trade name for nandrolone decanoate) at levels which were quite extraordinary. The dosages he initially used were supposedly Sustanon 250 milligrams per millilitre, twice a week (500 mg); Stanazole 160 milligrams per week and Decka 50 100 milligrams per week. Then after six weeks, his steroid regime was increased to Sustanon 800 milligrams per week and Stanazole increased to 320 milligrams per week.

As Mr Clarke-Saunders observed, this "amount of intravenous anabolic usage is sufficient to introduce a syndrome referred to as Steroid Rage."

Mr Jaafar's supposed steroid regime was 800 milligrams of Sustanon per week, which was some four times the top end of the recommended dosage. Stanazole increased to 320 milligrams per week which is just over twice the level used by athletes self-administering the drugs to improve sports performance. Even the Decka 50 at 100 milligrams per week was some three to four times the top end of the recommended dosage!! Clearly, this was a hefty regime of steroids – if it were true. These large dosage regimes of these steroids would lead to serious health problems, including oedema (fluid retention and bloating), suppression of clotting factors of the blood, elevated cholesterol (cholesterolemia), mood disorders and depression. It is more likely that these steroids were obtained illegitimately, of which the potency could be anyone's guess. Whilst prescription-only medicine undergoes strict quality control protocols outlined by the Therapeutic Goods Administration (TGA), 'street drugs' have no such controls, other than 'market forces'...

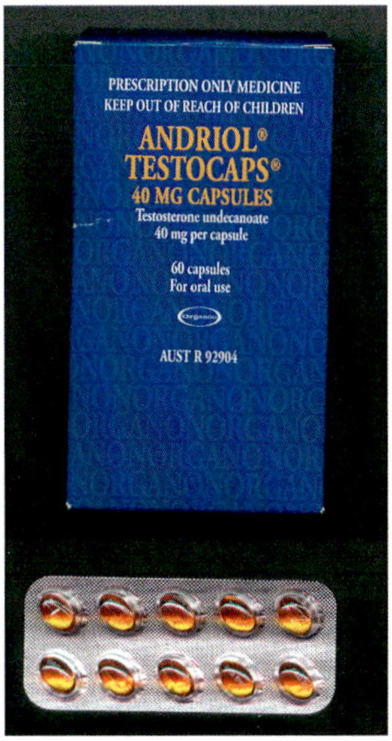


*Fig. 65: View of a legitimate pack of a steroid, shown here is 'Andriol' a brand of testosterone.*

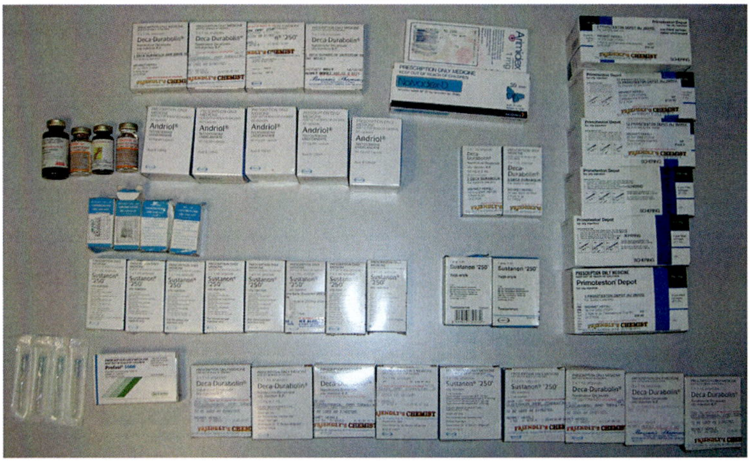

*Fig. 66: Steroids seized – some appear legitimate.*
*[Photos: Bass Hill Crime Scene, NSW Police Force]*

## On Trial for Armed Robbery

On 22 April 2005 Jamil Jaafar, stood trial in the NSW District Court for armed robbery at a Westpac Bank, Auburn on 20 December 2003.

Ms Natalie Olender was the Crown Prosecutor and Mr Andrew Bellanto QC appeared for the defence, Judge Hosking presided.

Mr Clarke-Saunders for the defence, was examined at length about the "amount of intravenous anabolic usage is sufficient to introduce a syndrome referred to as Steroid Rage." His Honour further questioned Mr Clarke-Saunders in relation to his steroid usage asking, "Just so that I understand this Mr Clark-Saunders, are you saying that this man had a serotonin deficiency?"

To which he replied, "It's a hypothesis. It's my experience that individuals, not at the time of the offences and preceeding the offences while he was consuming increasing amounts of anabolic steroids, yes, I would say yes to that question."

He was further questioned on this issue, "You've said in ... your report under the heading impulse control disorder. 'In relation to his psychological steroid addiction and associated rage is compounded by serotonin deficiency'."

His Honour, further asked, "The reason I ask you that question is that you seem to state that as a fact where as you are telling me that it is really an hypothesis. Is that correct?"

Clarke-Saunders' answer was: "That is my professional opinion."

Further questioning by legal counsel and His Honour centred around clinical depression, impulse control disorders and serotonin deficiencies supposedly, brought about Mr. Jaafar's steroid usage. One key question was, "Are you able to say then how you came to the conclusion that a precipitating factor to the offender's offending behaviour is one of steroid rage, if in fact you didn't take a history from the offender in relation to that use of anabolic steroids?"
Mr Clark-Saunders: "I incorporated research from the Internet from NIDA [National Institute on Drug Abuse] and also from research into anabolic steroids and the mind. Because what I concluded is that I reviewed the defendant's history and there was no evidence of criminality prior to these offences. Although he was suffering from depression there was no history of anti-social behaviour."

The subsequent evidence did not support this, and the quantities of steroids supposedly consumed were not supported by testimony. Where to now?

I was subsequently called, and cross examined by the defence. "Do you agree that steroid use can affect one's belief in oneself, affect one's behaviour, that type of thing, depending upon dosage?"

I had to agree, "Most definitely, but it depends upon dosage. At various high levels there is anecdotal evidence that it can cause mood changes in some folk." I was further questioned and explained the problems associated with steroid usage in particular, steroids being obtained on the black market.

"Being a black market trade, in some respects there is no control over purity?"

"No. Normally these type of steroids are broken down, with various types of [vegetable] oil. As I indicated [earlier] with peanut oil, for one example."

Further questioning sought to establish a link between steroid usage and rage.

I indicated that, “Rage by definition whether steroid induced or otherwise, is violent, uncontrollable anger.”

“You’ve indicated there from the fact sheet, that it doesn’t appear that the offender’s behaviour in relation to his role was that of any aggressive behaviour?”

I had to agree, and the amount and type of steroids he had supposedly taken appeared very unlikely. Given the likelihood of black market origins of the steroids – the purity would have been doubtful. There have been various reports and studies that suggest a link between anabolic steroid use and aggressive behaviour. However, a causal relationship has not yet been clearly established.

It may be that people who are potentially more aggressive would be more likely to use anabolic steroids. Currently, it appears that, despite reports of violent behaviour among steroid users, there is little scientific evidence that use of anabolic steroids actually causes aggression.

## Conclusion

It was unlikely that Jaafar was in a “steroid-induced rage compounded by a serotonin deficiency.” But it certainly was a novel defence! The robbery was carefully planned down to the last detail, the staff were carefully restrained with cable ties, Uniden handheld scanners were used, staff were threatened, taser stun guns and previous inside knowledge of banking practices were used to the robbers’ advantage. This was a well-organised and professional robbery. But for someone notifying the Police, and their rapid handling of the matter, it is probable the Jaafar and his accomplices would have escaped with a very large amount of stolen money.

During the course of the investigation a second weapon was located in the rear of a shopkeeper’s yard. This yard was along the route that the second offender Huang took on foot. Huang’s DNA profile was matched with the shoe and dust mask located. In order to secure a conviction Detective Beaumont went back to the canvass forms and managed to locate a shopkeeper who had witnessed a male running from the bank towards Coles. His description of the offender matched that of Huang, and he further indicated that he noticed the man was removing a white dust mask as he ran. This offender’s last location was put within a short distance of where the dust mask and shoe was found. Huang was charged with aggravated robbery’, for ‘depriving of a person’s liberty’, three counts of robbery in company and one count of ‘robbery and assault.’

Jaafar received a sentence of two years with a non-parole period of eighteen months.

Huang received a sentence of five years with a non-parole period of three years. Huang appealed against his conviction, but this was dismissed.

To date there is one offender outstanding. However, there is also one fingerprint outstanding that has yet to be matched from the scene, and numerous other prints from the exhibits examined that have not been identified.

# 9
# The Body in the Bin Murder

*"No good deed goes unpunished."*

Clare Booth Luce

## A Grisly Find

It was garbage night on a cool evening of June 29, 2003, when a Redfern resident made his grisly find – a human body protruding from a wheelie bin sitting on the kerb. The body had been dumped head first into a wheeled domestic bin at the corner of Renwick and James Streets, Redfern, an inner Sydney suburb, New South Wales.

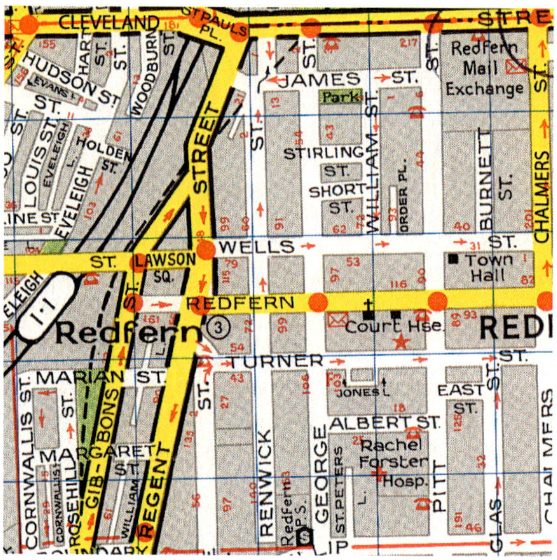


*Fig. 67: Map of Renwick and James Streets, Redfern, NSW.*

A resident, Mr Charles Pryor said he discovered the body about ten p.m. as he went to take out the rubbish after returning home.

He said, "Almost directly opposite the house there was a wheelie bin with an object sticking out of the top. I thought that I should check it out." He went on to say, "I extended my arm and felt around the object that was sticking out of the top and it felt soft and I felt that there was a body in there. It was unusual, because we don't have wheelie bins on that street."

**Police Summoned**

Quite alarmed at this point, Mr Pryor hurried back to his unit and called the police. They were on the scene about twenty minutes later and carefully dragged the body out of the bin. The deceased was found to have been dumped head first into the bin with his feet protruding at an odd angle from the top. A Caribee brand sleeping bag with the words underneath stating (ironically) “LIVE THE ADVENTURE” was covering the top half of the deceased up to the thigh and two black plastic garbage bags covered the deceased’s legs. Also found in the bin was a box of cornflakes, a meat tray, a pair of shoes… and, not surprisingly, a large amount of blood.

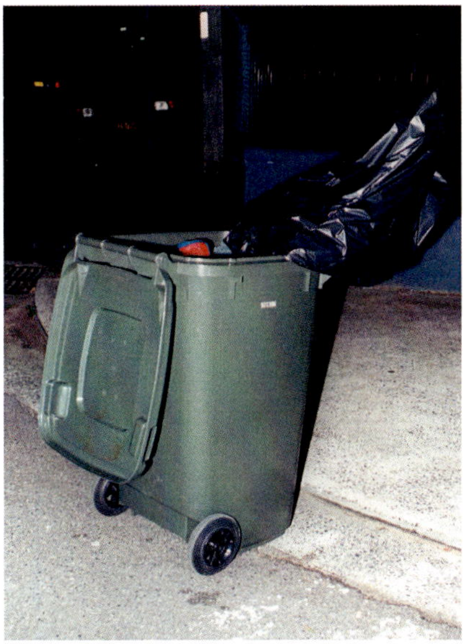

*Fig. 68: The wheelie bin as found by Mr Pryor*

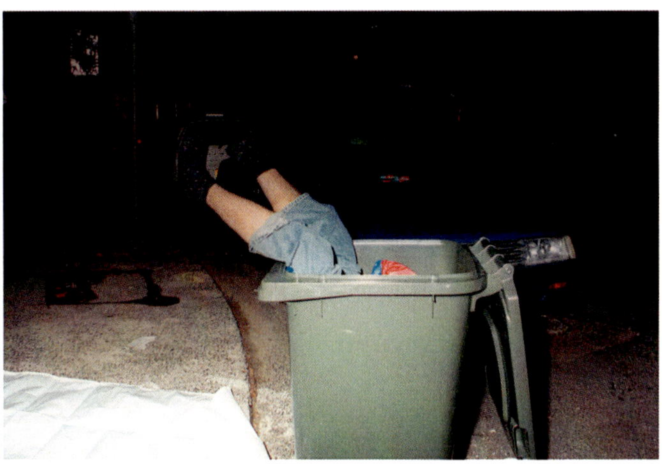

*Fig. 69: Deceased in the wheelie bin with plastic bags removed*

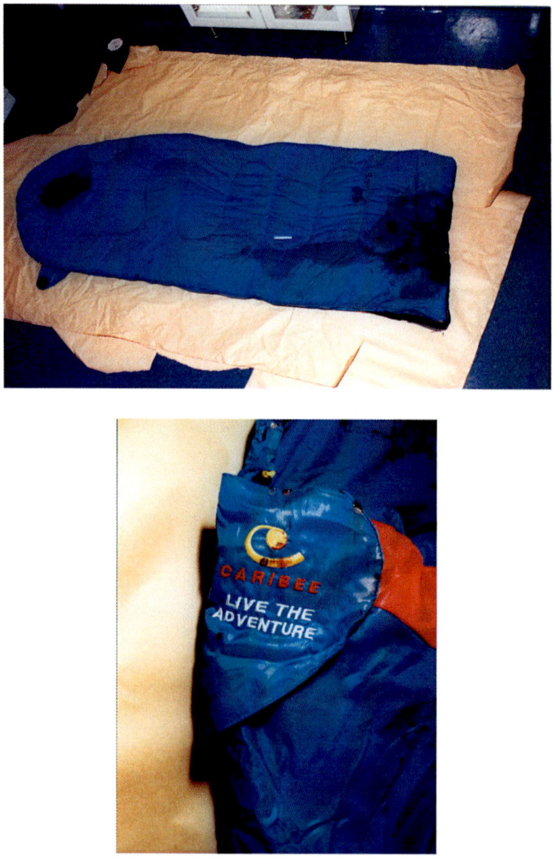


*Fig.70 a & b: The blood stained 'Caribee' sleeping bag, and below and the ironic logo: "Live the Adventure"*

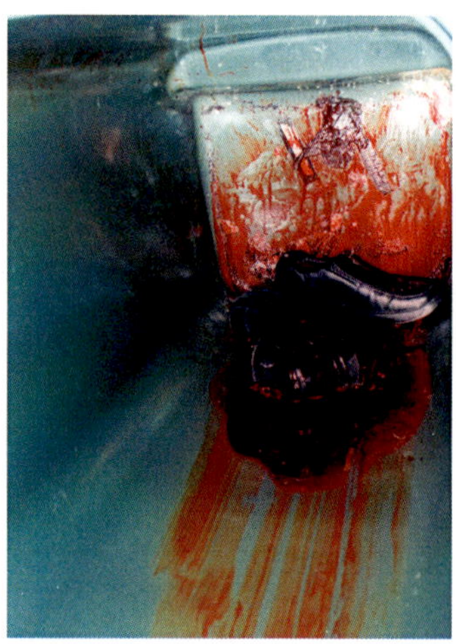

*Fig. 71: Shoes and blood in the wheelie bin.*
*[Photos: Redfern Crime Scene, NSW Police Force]*

## The Victim

A crime scene was established, and the cadaver was duly taken to the Glebe morgue for post mortem examination. While this was going on, a number of constables spent the night looking for clues as to how the man had died and (if possible) just when his body had been dumped in the wheelie bin.

After extensive enquiries by Redfern detectives, spanning some weeks, the body found in the wheelie bin was later identified as Shoukat Ali Mohammed, an Indian national. Shoukat Ali Mohammed, thirty-one years old, had arrived in Sydney, Australia from India in February, 1998 on a student visa.

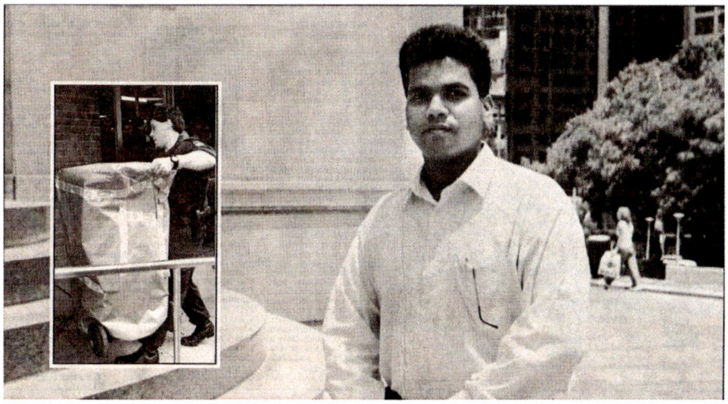

*Fig. 72: The victim Shoukat Ali Mohammed and wheelie bin insert.*
*Source:* Daily Telegraph.

He obtained casual work with a contract cleaning company Baggett and Markham Services, having last worked at the East Village Hotel on Palmer Street in Darlinghurst on the morning of 29 June, 2003.

## Fatal Liaison

Three years earlier in 2000 he met a fellow countryman, who I will call 'John Brown' for the purpose of this story, in the Surry Hills area. Brown had previously travelled from India to Australia in 1999. John Brown was introduced to the principals of Baggett and Markham Services, and subsequently filled in for Shoukat Mohammed when he was unable to attend work for various reasons. During 2002 John Brown shared a residence in Redfern with Youssef Tecle Imnetu, a Belgian national, also of Indian descent, known as Joe.

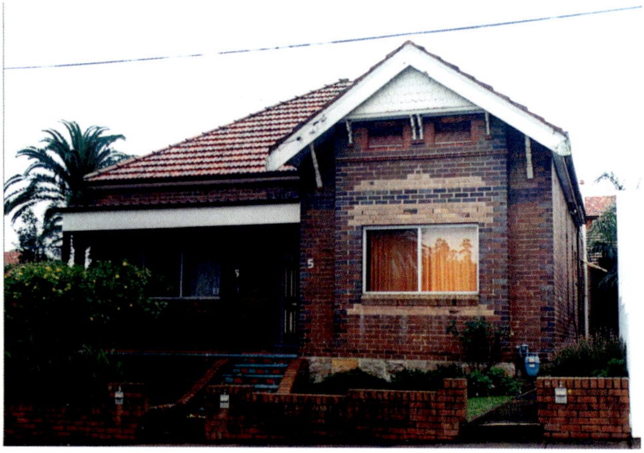

*Fig. 73: The house where Shoukat Ali Mohammed stayed while in Redfern, Sydney, NSW*

In 2003 Joe Imnetu moved into a two bedroom home unit 13/187 in Cleveland Street, Redfern sharing with others. Not surprisingly, John Brown was a regular visitor to the unit.

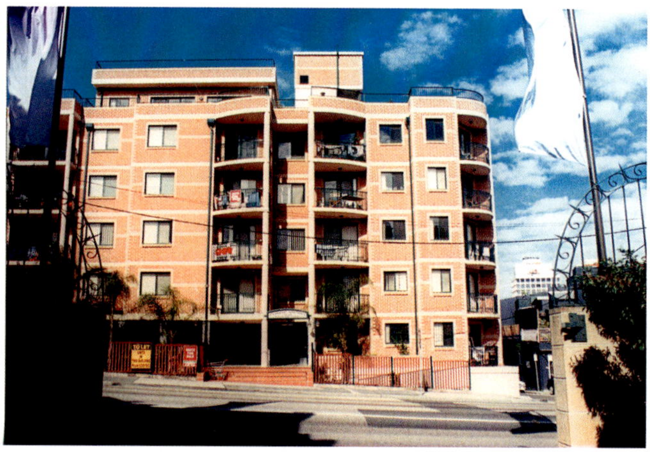

*Fig. 74: Block of units at 187 Cleveland Street, Redfern*

During this time, Shoukat Mohammed received $178,000 in settlement over a workplace injury. Several other people were aware of this windfall – especially John Brown, who persuaded his friend to give him $20,000 which he needed to pay for a bridging visa after his student visa had expired. At some point after this Joe Imnetu and John Brown had decided to engage in a criminal enterprise to murder Shoukat Mohammed and it appears more than likely that money was the prime motive. At about two p.m. in the afternoon of June 29, 2003 Shoukat Mohammed receives a call on his mobile from Joe Imnetu…

### Candid Security Camera

About two thirty p.m. that day a security camera recorded Shoukat Ali Mohammed's last movements as he arrived at the Cleveland Street units and afterwards parking his car in the underground car park. John Brown then joins him and they leave the car and enter the internal lift together. Later, at six fifty-nine p.m. the security camera records John Brown leaving the car park lift and leaving the building through a security roller door that opened onto Renwick Lane.

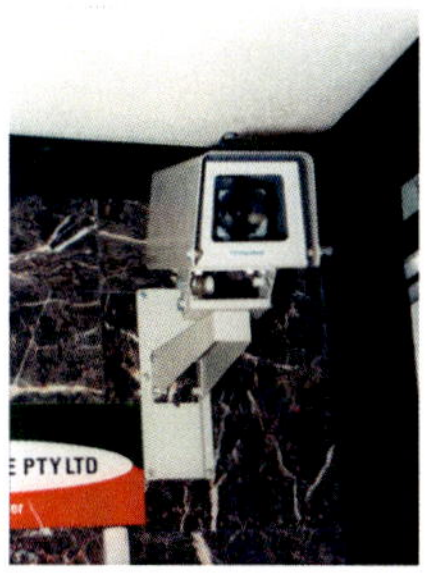


*Fig. 75: Security video camera installed in the unit building 'the ever seeing eye of the security camera'.*

Moments later, he re-enters with a wheelie bin which he takes to the lift. At eight fifteen p.m. John Brown and Joe Imnetu are recorded leaving the elevator.

Brown was seen pushing the wheelie bin with something dark protruding from the bin wrapped in black plastic, while Joe Imnetu walked in front of him.

Later, Brown and Imnetu were again recorded on security camera, entering Shoukat Mohammed's car and driving it from the car park. At ten p.m. that evening, Shoukat Ali Mohammed's lifeless body was found by Mr Pryor.

### Post Mortem

At the time of the post mortem, carried out by Doctor Paul Botterill, Department of Forensic Medicine, Glebe, was that the "cause of death was not completely clear and although the findings were accentuated by the positioning of the body in the wheelie bin, the features were consistent with strangulation."

Further investigations were then carried out. The toxicology report showed a blood morphine level of 0.2 milligrams per litre, as well as heroin (diacetylmorphine), monoacetylmorphine (a breakdown product of heroin) and acetylcodeine (an impurity which often occurs in 'street grade' heroin) was detected in the stomach contents. Users and/or addicts generally inject heroin, however, these latter results strongly suggested that the heroin had been consumed orally. Morphine and codeine were also detected in his urine, indicating Shoukat Mohammed had been alive for some time, hours maybe, after consuming the drug.

As heroin, an illicit drug, was involved it appeared prudent to eliminate the possibility that the victim was a drug user. A sample of his hair was forwarded onto the Victorian Institute of Forensic Medicine (VIFM) for analysis. Hair is a useful sample to test, because it can provide a 'drug history' of the deceased.

**Analytical Report from VIFM**

The results received however, showed no morphine or 6-monoacetylmorphine was detected, with only codeine being detected in the hair sample. If the deceased was a user of heroin, morphine and/or monoacetylmorphine this would have been detected in the deceased's hair sample, and if a regular user, possibly all three drugs would have been found. Codeine is present in a wide variety of pharmaceutical preparations, including cough mixtures.

Shoukat Mohammed clearly was not a regular user of heroin, and that the drug had most likely had been placed surreptitiously in a drink as "the stomach contained some turbid fluid." where heroin and its breakdown products were detected.

**Meanwhile 'Back at the Station'**

Joe Imnetu moved from 13/187 Cleveland Street, Redfern around July 6, 2003. Then, on July 17, 2003 John Brown left Australia on a Malaysian Airlines flight to New Delhi, India, having been deported for being in breach of his student visa. This occurred before his involvement in the crime became known. Just two days later, a search warrant was executed at the Cleveland Street address. Bloodstained carpet in the bedroom formerly occupied by Joe Imnetu and a piece of bloodstained electrical cord and switch were found. Mohammed had most likely had been murdered in this bedroom and Joe Imnetu had spent the last week (after the murder), sleeping in this room (number 13) before moving out. He was obviously not superstitious!

Police inquiries revealed that Joe Imnetu met with another person at Sydney Town Hall, Sydney where he apparently told this person that, 'Some people came into his unit, blindfolded him and told him to dispose of the body in the rubbish bin.'

Curiously, at about six twenty p.m. on the 1 August, 2003 Joe Imnetu attended Redfern Police Station where after revealing his participation in the crime.

He was arrested and interviewed. Initially, he said that he could not remember what he did on the 29 June, later changing his version stating John Brown and Shoukat Ali Mohammed had in fact attended 13/187 Cleveland Street, Redfern at about two p.m. that day. He went out with John Brown in the afternoon and left the victim alone in the unit. He further said that he left about ten p.m. and returned about midnight and then went to sleep. At no stage did he go to the basement car park on the 29 June, even though the security footage clearly showed otherwise. Joe Imnetu's new address at 4/83 Old South Head Road,

Bondi Junction was subsequently searched and, very incriminating a black top with the insignia "DKNY" on the front was found.

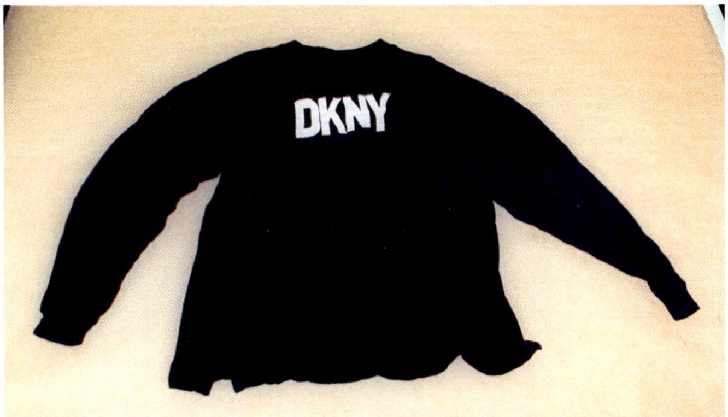


*Fig. 76: The incriminating 'DKNY' top.*

This top was worn by Imnetu in the video footage as the victim was being wheeled out in the garbage bin!

**On Trial for Murder**

On June 14 2005, Youssef Tecle Imnetu alias Joe Imnetu, a twenty-four-year–old Belgian national, stood trial in the NSW Supreme Court for the slaying of Shoukat Ali Mohammed on June 29, 2003. Crown Prosecutor Dan Howard SC, said that the two men, Joe Imnetu and his flatmate John Brown, were observed on security video footage in their apartment building, taking a wheelie bin with something protruding from it shortly after Shoukat Mohammed was believed to have been murdered.

"The cameras then show there is something protruding from the bin wrapped in black plastic," he said.

A post mortem examination revealed that Shoukat Mohammed had been orally overdosed on heroin, hit with a blunt object and then strangled.

Mr Howard said, "I'll be calling the evidence of a number of people who knew the deceased," and "this evidence will show he was not a drug user."

I was previously summonsed to Mr Howard's office and advised that the analysis of the deceased's hair would confirm one way or another whether he was a drug user, especially heroin.

The analytical report confirmed my beliefs about the victim, and I expressed that in court. He was not a regular drug user, and certainly not into heroin. However, it appeared he was also bludgeoned with a baseball bat before his body was stuffed into a wheelie bin. Actually, all three methods could have resulted in his death.

## Sentence

On August 26, 2005 Joe Imnetu appeared for sentencing after a jury found him guilty of the murder of Shoukat Ali Mohamed. He was subsequently jailed for a minimum of twenty years for the murder.

**20 years jail for wheelie bin murder**

A SYDNEY court yesterday jailed a man for a minimum 20 years for the murder of an Indian man whose body was dumped in a wheelie bin.

Belgian national Youssef Tecle Imnetu, 24, appeared for sentencing after a jury found him guilty of the murder of Shoukat Ali Mohamed in inner-city Redfern on June 29, 2003.

The Supreme Court was told that Imnetu and a flatmate force-fed Mr Mohamed heroin and struck him over the head with a baseball bat, before strangling him and dumping his body in a wheelie bin outside their Cleveland St apartment block.

The flatmate, Basheeruddin Mohamed, also known as Ben, allegedly owed Mohamed $20,000.

Before his involvement in Mr Mohamed's murder was known, Ben was deported for being in breach of his student visa.

*Fig. 77: This paragraph subsequently appeared in the Sydney Morning Herald.*

## Conclusion

Without a doubt, the prime motive for this appalling murder had to be greed. When the orally ingested heroin did not seem to be working on the victim, more drastic measures were utilised with a deadly outcome. It was a shocking payback to a friend and, if it had not been for an alert local resident checking out the wheelie bin with its grisly contents, they may well have got away with a premeditated murder.

Further, and thanks to advice and tip-offs from the victim's relatives, the other villain: 'John Brown' aka Ben Driscoll or Basheeruddin Mohamed was apprehended in India and he was sent back to Australia to face trial – and subsequently joined his accomplice in gaol!

# 10
# Death of a Drug Dealer: the Ecstasy and Agony!

*"There are only three sins – causing pain, causing fear and causing anguish. The rest is window dressing."*

Roger Caras

## Introduction

'Ecstasy' is a very popular drug of abuse. Following cannabis and amphetamines, MDMA is the third most widely used illicit drug in Australia. This case involved a drug dealer who enjoyed regular drug usage including Ecstasy in addition to selling a variety of other drugs at some considerable profit, and the subsequent consequences of enforcing his 'authority' while under the influence of the drugs. This time he clearly got in over his head, costing him the ultimate price.

## Paying a Visit

It was a drizzly early morning after midnight on 11 March 2003, when David Hudson, aged forty-four, a known drug dealer, drove up to the premises of Sean Galgey at 490 Beach Road at Batehaven, Batemans Bay. The night and the weather conditions were certainly not auspicious, with further heavy rain on the way. But it was debt-collection time for some drug money and Sean Galgey owed him $1000. Time for payment! In the meantime, another customer of Hudson, David Florit was brokering a repayment which was to be in the form of money and/or sexual favours by Sean Galgey's girlfriend. As you do, but this was a drug dealer's world, and deals are settled in various ways.

Soon after the arrival of Hudson, a heated argument broke out between the three males regarding the drug debt. There appeared to be no room for negotiation.

Unfortunately, the argument became loud and aggressive with threats being made against all persons present. At one stage, Hudson attempted to punch both Florit and Galgey, and at one time chased Galgey down the road. Galgey returned and the argument and fighting continued. Hudson then removed his shirt and trousers apart from a pair of boxer shorts, and then proceeded to dance in an aggressive manner in the front yard of the property. This stance continued for sometime, with Hudson becoming very loud and more aggressive. Galgey shouted, "He's gone berserk!"A violent fight then broke out between the three males.

## The Showdown

It is not known exactly how the violent fight occurred between the three males. But what is known is that David Florit took a headlock on David Hudson, which was severe enough for both parties to fall to the ground.

Florit then screamed out, "Knock him unconscious!"

Galgey commenced to kick Hudson between the legs and to the stomach area, as well as punching him repeatedly.

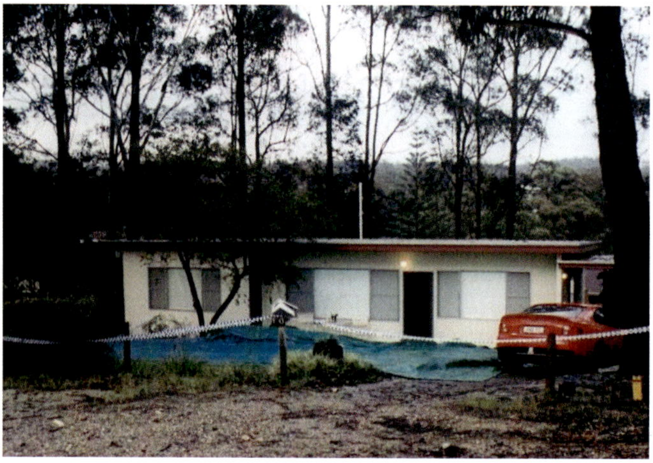

*Fig. 78: Crime scene where the incident occurred.*

## "Quick, Get the Baseball Bat!"

Galgey then ran into the house and got a baseball bat from the laundry. He then returned to where Hudson was being held by Florit. In an act of extraordinary brutality, he began hitting the restrained Hudson with the weapon a number of times. In the meantime, the now victim's legs were bound with a belt taken from the trousers he had removed. In addition, he was also bound by a bedsheet gathered from inside the house.

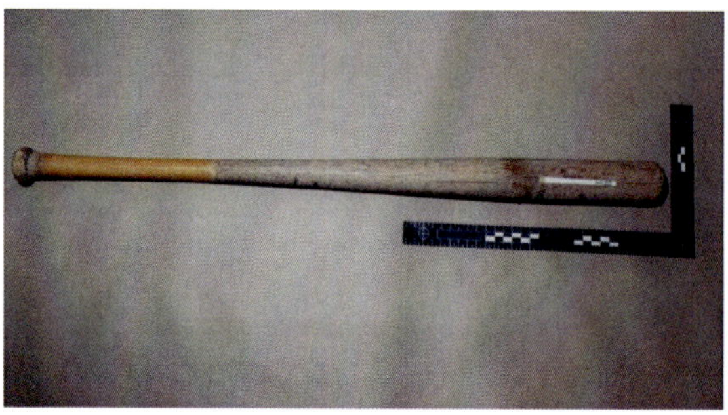

*Fig. 79: Baseball bat used in the attack*

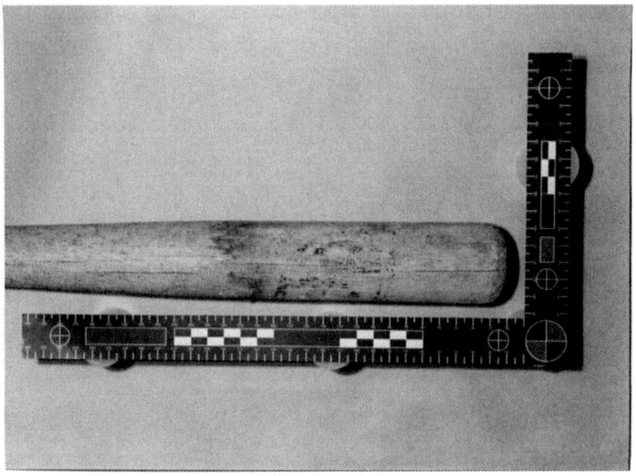

*Fig. 80: Close up of the bat showing blood stains*
*[Photos: Batemans' Bay Crime Scene, NSW Police Force]*

The beatings continued until Hudson lapsed in unconsciousness. By now a member in the house, who saw what was going on, had notified Bateman's Bay Police. Senior Constable Ken Cropper and Senior Constable O'Neill arrived at the scene and found Florit sitting on Hudson. Both Florit and Hudson were now soaked, as it was now raining heavily.

Florit spoke to them saying: "He's crazy. Watch him. He's dangerous. He was trying to kill us. He's high on speed. He's the most wanted man in New South Wales."

Senior Constable Cropper said, "Okay. Get off him."

He started to handcuff Hudson given Forit's outburst, when he realised Hudson was lying unconscious on the lawn.

"Are you okay?"

He wasn't …

**Crime Scene Blues**

Hudson was unresponsive to any questions from the attending police officers and his face was turning blue. The handcuffs were put away and the officer commenced expired air resuscitation. Further police arrived and cardio-pulmonary resuscitation (CPR) was commenced. CPR was continued until an ambulance arrived to take Hudson to Bateman's Bay Hospital. Meanwhile Florit was wandering around the crime scene clearly searching for something and he said, "Excuse me, I know youse are busy, but could I borrow your torch? I've lost my wallet in the front yard somewhere."

Senior Constable Garten said, "Your wallet is not a priority at the moment, this guy is more important."

Florit then replied, "It's got six hundred dollars in it!"

Senior Constable Garten replied, "We can't lend you the torch, the police are trying to save his life."

Florit was unhappy with this response, and became agitated when police would not help him to find his wallet – given the circumstances!

Forit walked away for a moment and turned, saying, "I hope he dies, he's a piece of shit."

Additional police arrive including Detective Sergeant Ed Freeman and Detective Senior Constable Clayton to carry out further the inquiries. Detective Sergeant Ed Freeman then asks, "What's happened here?"

Galgey replies, "It was self-defence, we had to protect ourselves, don't worry about it, it's all over drugs."

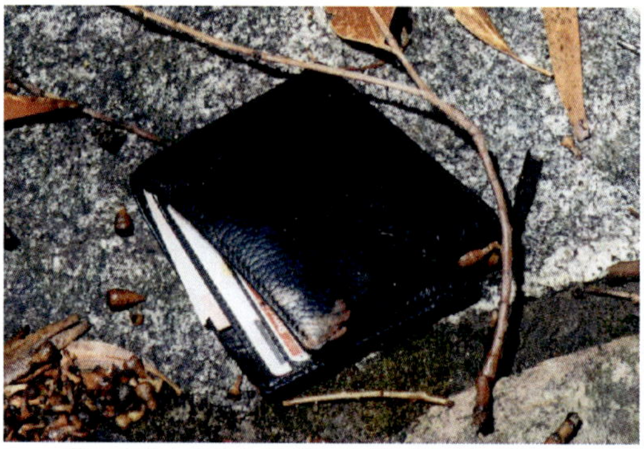

*Fig. 81: Offender's wallet at the scene*

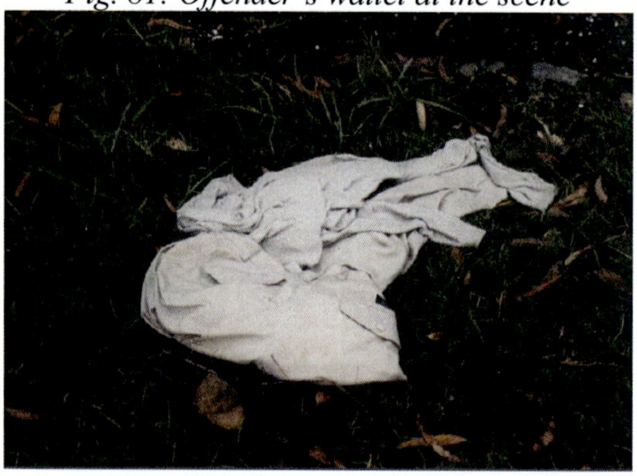

*Fig. 82: The victim's clothing*

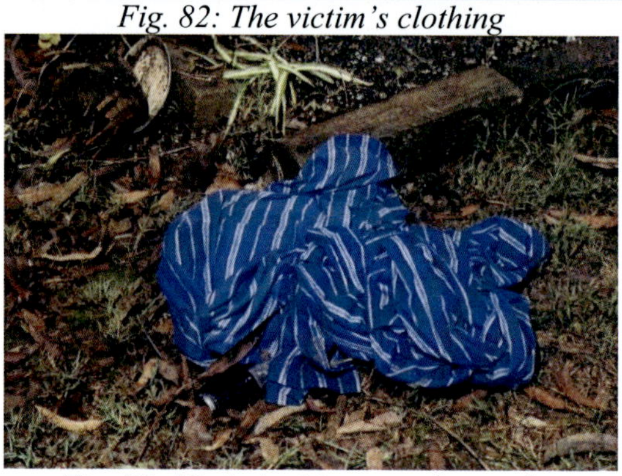

*Fig. 83: Victim's shirt near the garden*
*[Photos: Batemans' Bay Crime Scene, NSW Police Force]*

The area was subsequently covered by a tarpaulin, to protect the crime scene from the rain as it had now set in, and Florit and Galgey were taken back to Bateman's Bay Police station for questioning. It had been a tough, damp, violent night…

Hudson was subsequently transported to Bateman's Bay Hospital in a critical condition. As his condition further deteriorated, he was later transferred to Canberra Hospital where he died about midday on 12 March, 2003 the following day.

**Blood Levels Found**

According to the Analyst Certificate (ACT Government Analytical Laboratory report), blood samples taken from Hudson's body at post mortem were found to contain MDMA 0.68 milligrams per litre, methylamphetamine 0.14 milligrams per litre, citalopram 0.16 milligrams per litre, cannabis and its major metabolite (delta-9-THC acid) was also detected.

The blood sample taken from Hudson at post mortem showed a particularly high concentration of MDMA, well outside the therapeutic range (0.1 – 0.35 mg/L) for the drug, along with an elevated level of methylamphetamine – and this was some eleven hours and a half hours after the altercation. [Of the other drugs present, citalopram (an anti-depressant drug) was within the therapeutic range (0.048-0.243 mg/L), and cannabis was detected, indicating previous usage.]

Taken superficially, these amphetamines appeared to account for Hudson's very aggressive behaviour and possibly contributed to his demise.

**Post mortem**

However, the post mortem told quite a different story. Hudson had received a very severe hiding from a variety of sources. Bruising to the neck – apparently from a headlock, as well as numerous bruises to his upper torso, liver and kidney areas, groin and lower body from punching, kicking during the altercation – and more seriously, from the very liberal use of the baseball bat.

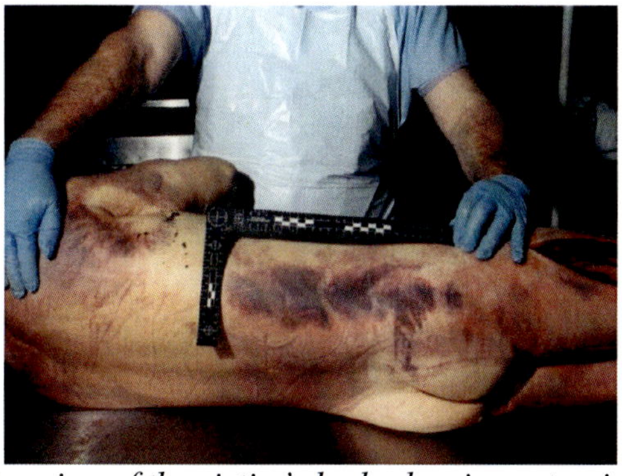

*Fig. 84: Overview of the victim's body showing extensive bruising.*

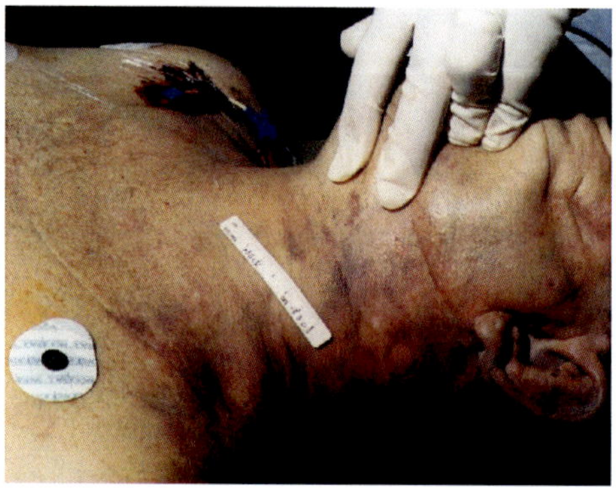

*Fig.85: Extensive bruising to neck.*
*[Photos: Batemans' Bay Crime Scene, NSW Police Force]*

Actually, some twenty-five injuries were identified on Hudson's corpse, the more serious of which were found around the deceased's main organs.

Forensic Pathologist Dr Malcolm Dodd described part of his examination as, "Serial sectioning of the liver [that] discloses a large blood-filled cavity within the central part of the right lobe... The cavity contains clotted blood with areas of lamination."

His liver had been seriously damaged.

"Examination of the retroperitoneal soft tissues discloses extensive acute haemorrhage within the right retroperitoneal potential space extending from the diaphragm to the inferior pole of the right kidney. The left retroperitoneal soft tissues are exceedingly oedematous but showed no evidence of haemorrhage." Hudson's kidneys had also been damaged.

The right-side kidney apparently fared worse than the left. Metabolism, storage and elimination are three mechanisms whereby the body ultimately removes drugs from their sites of action. Removal of drugs such as MDMA/ Ecstasy and methamphetamine, for example via the liver, kidneys and biliary system, accounts for most of the drug elimination. If any of these organs are damaged through various reasons, (disease etc.) then their efficiency is greatly reduced. An inefficient or damaged renal secretory mechanism will result in the build-up of drugs in the blood to potentially toxic levels. These damaged excretory organs involved in metabolism and elimination suggest a more likely explanation for the elevated levels of MDMA and methamphetamine levels detected in Hudson's blood, after a number of hours from the altercation.

I attended Bateman's Bay Court for the initial hearing, and gave evidence as to the levels of drugs found in Hudson's blood. I was concerned that a potentially toxic level of MDMA was found in his blood after so many hours. It just did not seem to add up.

In patients who had died of MDMA toxicity, the blood levels ranged from 0.110 to 1.26 milligrams per litre. Hudson's blood level of MDMA at 0.68 milligrams per litre, which was in the median of this range. It had to be due to his injuries and, in particular, damage to those vital metabolic and excretory organs:

his liver and kidneys. Essentially, the various organs ability to metabolise any drugs had been severely compromised. Part of my final statement ran, "that the presence of 3,4-methylenedioxymethamphetamine (or MDMA) most likely contributed to his observed behaviour at the time of the incident." And there the matter appeared to end.

However, some years later…

### A Very Unexpected Result

The matter appeared to have 'gone quiet' for some time. There were no good guys in this scenario. And so, the end result was even more unexpected. The matter had since moved from Bateman's Bay to Nowra District Court. Whilst, the dealer had a very poor criminal record, the final decision was very surprising. On the first day of the trial the Department of Public Prosecutions (DPP) decided, 'No Billed' (insufficient evidence for a successful prosecution) the matter without any witnesses giving evidence.

The DPP did not think that they would be able to prove that the assault/s by Galgey and Florit appeared to have caused the death of Hudson. The same defence being that the drugs in Hudson's system caused his death, not the assault – and the guy/s who beat the dealer to death, walked free!

# 11
# Suicide on the Farm

*"While we are focusing on fear, worry or hate, it is not possible for us to be experiencing happiness, enthusiasm or love."*

Bo Bennett

## A 'blue' and he 'shoots through'

Another case with which I had some involvement was the unfortunate death of a farmer by the suicidal ingestion of an arsenic formulation resulting in his death.

George Wiley and his wife Lucy (not their real names) had been married for some twenty-four years and despite some problems, appeared to have a relatively good marriage. However, one particular evening in late March 2004 proved to be exceptional. George had been drinking beer and Jack Daniels, a practice he would carry out about five times a week – and more than often than not, would get drunk. He mostly drank at the Royal Hotel (so many country towns in Australia have 'Royal Hotels'!) and at the end of the night go home and then head for bed. George's wife Lucy, a school teacher, arrived home at about five p.m. George arrived about half an hour later. After asking about each other's day and further pleasant conversation. Lucy then asked George about some money that was missing from the drawer which was going to be used to pay people who had worked on the farm the previous weekend. George then became defensive and began to argue with his wife about the money. Apparently, they regularly argued about money but this issue, apparently, touched a nerve.

He then told his wife, "Well, piss off and go to your meeting." Adding, "If you reckon I spend money, watch me now."

Lucy left, as she had a "year seven parents meet the teachers night", where they have an informal get-together to discuss a pupil's educational progress with their parents.

Lucy returned home about nine p.m. to nine thirty p.m.

Her husband's car was not there and assuming he had gone back "to the pub, more than likely the Royal Hotel." After a fitful night she awoke at seven thirty a.m., and her husband was still not at home, "Could he have stayed at the Royal Hotel for the night?" she thought. This was totally out of "the ordinary" for George.

Lucy reflected, "Could he have stayed at the farmhouse for the night?" Lucy then went to work, signed on and went to her office. She then started working on her computer and then went to the school's morning assembly. Lucy then attended a further meeting, which concluded about 10.05am. She then approached the Deputy Principal, informing she had some domestic problems and needed time off to sort out family problems.

Her request was granted and she left the school about 10.20am. Firstly, she went to their home in town, however George was not there. Lucy then grabbed some gum-boots, as previous rain made it difficult to enter the property without them, and drove to the property. She drove to the property about 10.30am and found the gates to the property still open.

As she entered the property, George's dogs came running up to Lucy's car. George's car was parked beside the farmhouse. It was then that she noticed the passenger's door was open…

**Down on the farm a body is found**

George was found hanging out of the car and at the time was thought to be asleep.

Lucy was first on the scene and, "I thought he was just drunk and fell asleep and was hanging out the car asleep."

As she got up closer to the car, she noticed that he was a strange colour and positioned at a weird angle.

"He was sort of a purple-grey colour from his neck to his head, however around his waist he was a white colour. His pants had slipped down a bit around his waist and it looked like his body had stretched longer than what it was usually.

"I also saw that there was some blood coming from his nose and had dripped down his moustache … When I touched him he was just so cold. I began screaming, 'No! No! No!'".

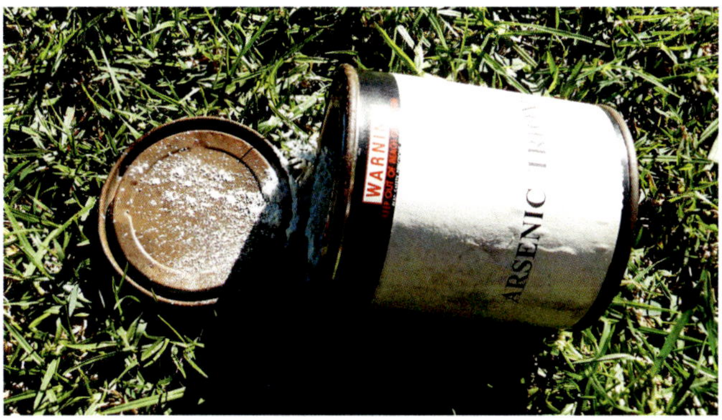


*Fig. 87: Can of Arsenic Trioxide found at the scene.*

Lucy had to get back to the high school where she could get help from someone she could trust. The ambulance and Police were contacted. George had, unfortunately, passed away sometime earlier… Possible money problems?

So, why did George do himself in? Police questioned Lucy at some length as to their financial situation.

She answered that their "Our current financial position is a position what I believe to be quite good. We own the farm outright on Chifley Lane… We own our house outright at Warrior Street… I am employed at Wee Waa High School where I earn approximately $60,000."

Lucy then further expanded on their financial situation… "The 2003/2004 summer yield of grapes was not as successful as what we had hoped for. This was due to the poor weather conditions that we endured this year. Our expenditure/debt is often the basis of arguments, however there is no major problems amongst us about debt…" So, there appeared to be no financial reason for George to take his own life.

So, why did he do it..?

## Toxicology and Post Mortem results

A blood sample taken at the post mortem showed the presence of 5.05 milligrams per litre of arsenic. The average arsenic levels found in blood due to intentional or accidental overdosage is 3.3 milligrams per litre [range: 0.6-9.3 mg/L]

He had clearly ingested sufficient of the toxin to do its destructive work, resulting in his death. An additional blood sample taken from George at post mortem showed a blood concentration of venlafaxine 0.3 milligrams and alcohol 0.108 grams per decilitre (100 millilitres of blood). Venlafaxine ('Effexor') is an antidepressive drug which works by inhibiting the re-uptake of certain neurotransmitters, including serotonin and adrenaline in the brain – and hopefully, maintaining the brain chemistry so that these levels can be maintained. Unfortunately, alcohol at elevated levels, can interfere with these desired outcomes…

The post mortem results showed that "His face shows bruising to upper and lower eyelids. Conjectiva [sic] multiple haemorrhage to both eyes. Some blood clotted around mouth and nose. Multiple bruising to neck (front) shoulders and both arms. Cyanosis of both ears… Fingernails cynanosis… Toenails cynanosis.

Furthermore that the, "Back of tongue very blue and congested. Larynx shows multiple small haemorrhages in the area of the larynx and on vocal cords. No evidence of obstruction."

## A Sad End

It was a sad end for George – and for his wife who truly cared for him. Unlike a lot of other cases I have encountered, George was in an apparently stable loving relationship, but he also suffered from depression. Hence, the need for venlafaxine. Unfortunately, being a farmer, he also had access to a very effective poison, arsenic, which he subsequently ingested with a quantity of alcohol, after an argument with his wife – with fatal consequences. This was a particularly sad end as there was really no worthwhile motive or reason for George's far too early demise…

# 12
# Up in Smoke

*"Fire is a good servant but a fearsome master."*

Anonymous

## Introduction

Deaths by fire are generally accidental, and suicide by this method is extremely rare. Self-immolation, also known as self-incineration, occurs when a person pours a flammable liquid generally petrol (or gasoline) onto themselves and setting it on fire. This has occurred in three victim categories: those with psychiatric problems, personal reasons or political motivations. However, when a fire is deliberately set, the case may be classified as homicide. When a body is found in the debris of a fire, it is essential to discover whether it was alive at the time and died of asphyxiation, or whether it was already dead and the fire was started to conceal a murder. Samples of blood from the corpse are taken at post mortem. If they reveal the presence of carbon monoxide, it is almost certain that the victim was still breathing when the fire was started. The presence of soot particles in the airways and lungs is another positive indication.

In this particular case, it appears the deceased was still alive when the fire broke out…

## The Body in the Burnt-Out Van

It was the early hours of the morning, about three forty-five a.m. on Christmas Day 2002, in the Sydney suburb of Kellyville, that the body of an adult male was found lying prone in the footwell behind the front seats of a Tarago burnt-out van. The body had been extensively burnt with some areas of skin visible in an unburnt condition on the front of his body. The body of the deceased was clothed in the remnants of a burnt white polo shirt and burnt black trackpants. The soles of the shoes were present on the corpse's feet but were fused to the door and came off the feet when the door of the van was opened.

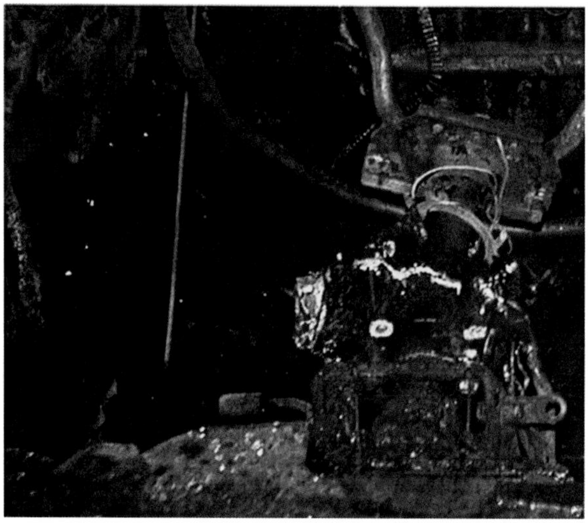

*Fig. 88: Burnt out interior of the van-front view*

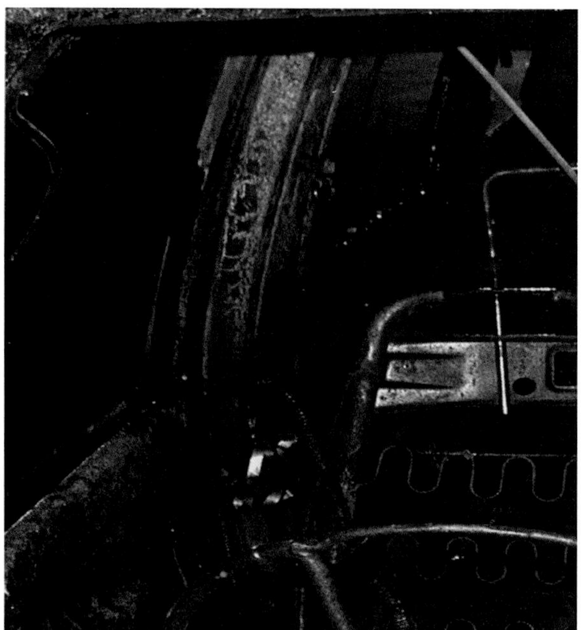

*Fig. 89: Burnt out interior of the van – side view*

When the body was removed from the van it was in a pugilistic position, its fists clenched in the characteristic posture of a boxer. This is typical of burn victims as the muscles in their arms seize up through the heat of the fire.

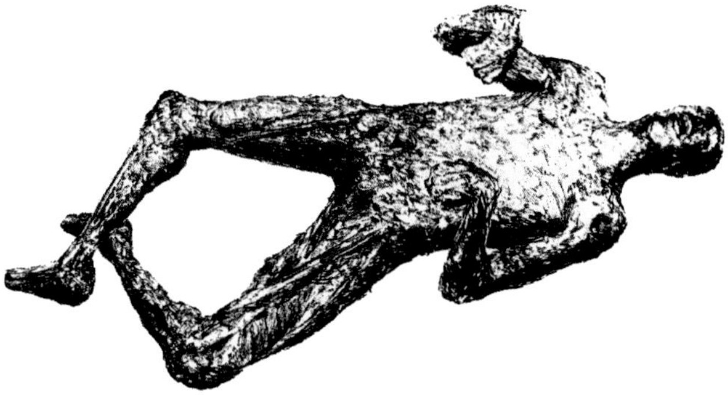

*Fig. 90: A typical pugilistic position of a burn victim.*

The back of his body was burnt and his front appeared covered with soot with areas of unburnt skin. A cherry-red fluid exuded from his mouth. This could have been due to a number of things including, most likely, carbon monoxide poisoning.

**Toxicology and Post Mortem results**

A blood sample taken at the post mortem showed the presence of delta-9-THC 0.008 milligrams per litre and delta-9-THC acid 0.016 milligrams per litre. In addition, his blood alcohol level was 0.249 grams per decilitre (100 millilitres) of blood. This combination would have been sufficient to render him in a very deep sleep, if not comatose. Cannabis also exacerbates the effects of alcohol.

Further, the carbon monoxide level was found to be 63% saturation, which would have been sufficient to result in his death. At a blood saturation of carbon monoxide of 50 to 60%, unconsciousness and coma with intermittent convulsions results. At a blood saturation of 60 to 70 % carbon monoxide, coma with intermittent convulsions is observed, depressed heart action and respiration and death are very likely. Carbon monoxide is present or produced whenever carbon-containing material is incompletely oxidised, as in burning material in a confined space such as a vehicle with insufficient draft. The haemoglobin in the blood combines with carbon monoxide (forming carboxyhaemoglobin) 200 to 300 times as readily as it does with oxygen and dissociates from it 250 times as slowly. The symptoms produced by carbon monoxide poisoning range from headache and dizziness to unconsciousness and death. The progression in severity is in accordance with the increase in the percent of saturation of haemoglobin with carbon monoxide in the air breathed and duration of exposure. At a blood saturation of carbon monoxide of 63 % – along with the alcohol level and cannabis present – death was pretty much certain, aside from the burns sustained from severe respiratory depression.

# 13
# Drink Spiking: A Two-Man 'Crime Wave'

*"Each betrayal begins with trust."*

Phish

## Introduction

Drink spiking has been carried out for many years beginning with the infamous 'Micky Finn' where the drug chloral hydrate was originally used, and even featured in the James Bond film *From Russia with Love.* Since then a large number of drugs have been used for this insidious crime including 'Rohypnol' (flunitrazepam). This drug featured so frequently in various drug-facilitated sexual assaults (DFSAs) that it became known as the 'date-rape drug'. The authorities (Therapeutic Goods Authority (TGA), in particular) placed restrictions on the use of these drugs. However, predatory drink-spikers are always 'on the prowl' and the anti-convulsant drug, clonazepam, apparently slipped through the regulatory net.

Unfortunately, this drug has been implicated in a number of other DFSA cases prior to this matter, but not on this scale…

**Drink-spiking horror**

**Women 'drugged, raped and robbed'**

By VIVA GOLDNER
Court Reporter

SORDID details of an alleged drink-spiking spree were revealed yesterday, with two men accused of drugging 12 people at popular city venues.

Posing as friendly strangers, Chebli Djait and Adel Samadi shouted their victims drinks, coffee or lunch over six days in October last year, Central Local Court heard.

But their charms allegedly masked evil intent, with the two men accused of raping three women and stealing thousands of dollars worth of cash and property from their young victims.

Djait, of Peakhurst, and Samadi, of Belmore, yesterday faced a committal hearing on several charges of using a stupefying drug with intent to steal, having - sexual intercourse without consent and receiving stolen goods.

The court heard most of the victims were approached while they drank in groups at the Three Wise Monkeys bar on George St, The Shark Hotel on Liverpool St or Darling Harbour's Pontoon Bar.

Djait and Samadi allegedly slipped the drug Clonazepam — marketed by Roche as Rivotril and used to treat epilepsy — into drinks bought for 10 women and two men.

Three women were allegedly sexually assaulted while property including cameras, mobile phones, a watch and wallets with cash and credit cards were stolen from others.

In a statement tendered to the court, a 24-year-old Korean student detailed her harrowing ordeal after meeting the two accused on October 17 at the Shark Hotel.

The strangers introduced themselves as "Andy" and "Dylan" from New Caledonia and shouted three rounds of drinks.

"I had a Midori and pineapple . . . while we are talking I lost my memory. I don't remember leaving the hotel," she said.

She woke the next morning and recalls just snatches of the alleged ensuing attacks.

"My eyes were open but I could not see properly. I couldn't think properly. I couldn't resist. He took off my underwear," she said.

She spent most of the day in a drugged sleep, and was assaulted three times by the accused, the court heard.

Another victim, a 22-year-old Japanese tourist, said she did not recall leaving The Three Wise Monkeys bar, but woke the next morning in bed with the man she knew as "Andy".

The hearing continues today.

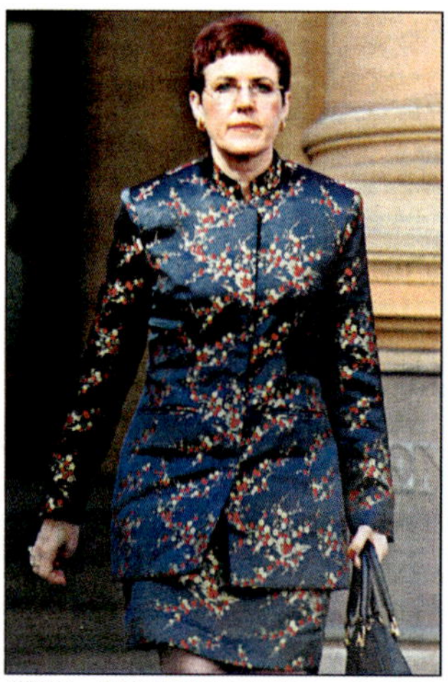

Witness . . . Susan Alexander yesterday. *Picture: GARY RAMAGE*

**'You wouldn't even taste it'**

VICTIMS of a prescription drug allegedly used in a spate of spikings would not know of its presence, an expert told the court.

The effects of anti-epileptic medication Clonazepam were revealed by Susan Alexander, head of regulatory affairs at Roche, which markets the drug as Rivotril.

Clonazepam belongs to a family of drugs which also includes Rohypnol — notorious for its abuse by predatory drink-spikers.

Rohypnol now contains a dye to warn of its presence in drinks, but Clonazepam would not change colour or taste of the liquid, Ms Alexander said.

Unlike Rohypnol, Ms Alexander said prior to this ongoing case there had not been evidence that Rivotril was being used as a "substance of abuse".

Ms Alexander told the court yesterday that clinical tests showed the Rivotril often had a sedative effect.

This was increased if the drug was taken with alcohol, she added.

*Fig. 91: Paper headline "Drink-spiking horror'*
*Source:* The Daily Telegraph*, July 28, 2005*

## A 'New Drug on the Block'

Clonazepam ('Rivotril', 'Paxam') is a benzodiazepine drug that has be used as an anticonvulsant to treat generalised epilepsy in adults and children, as well as restless legs syndrome and acute mania. It has marked sedative effects. Tolerance to the anti-epileptic effects tends to develop rather fast, which has limited its use for this complaint. This drug is a potent sedative and has been used as a substitute for flunitrazepam ('Rohypnol'). Clonazepam is generally administered in daily oral maintenance doses of 1.5 to 20 milligrams, in the form of 0.5-2 milligram tablets. Unfortunately, the drug does not change colour or taste of the liquid. It can in non-tolerant persons, result in central nervous system (CNS) depression including impaired alertness, transient amnesia, memory impairment and somnolence (sleepiness), these effects are exacerbated if alcohol is also consumed...

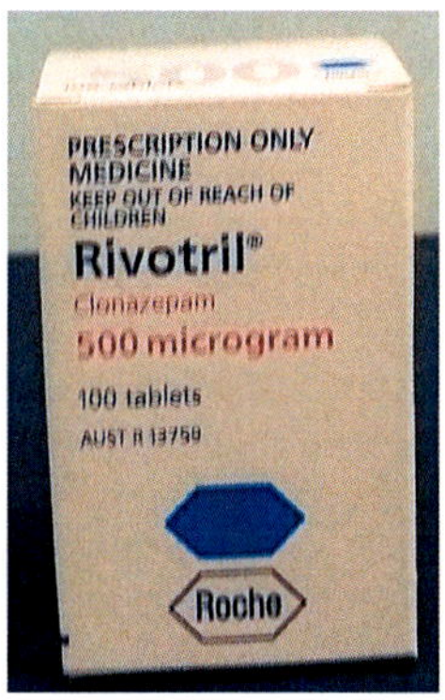


*Fig. 92: A typical pack of 'Rivotril'*

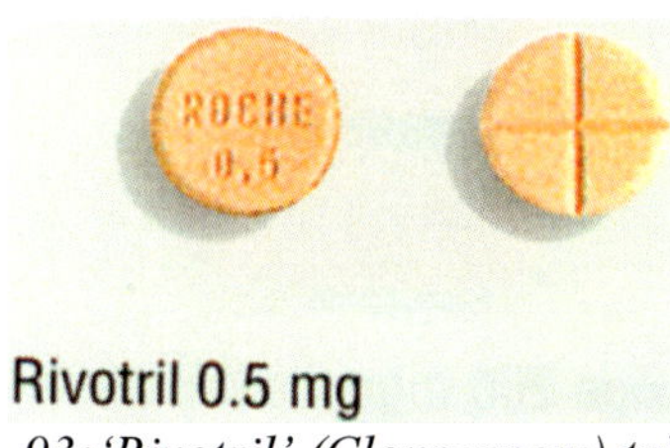


*Fig. 93: 'Rivotril' (Clonazepam) tablets*

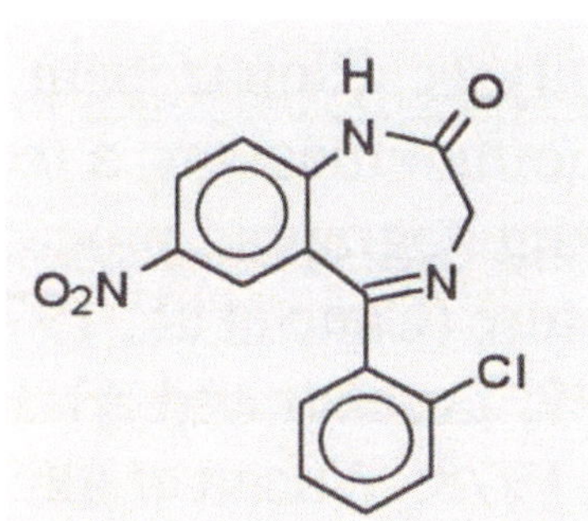

*Fig. 94: Chemical structure of clonazepam*

**Drink Spiking Rampage**

Chebli Djait and Adel Samadi who used alias names of 'Andy' and 'Dylan' worked together to spike the drinks of twelve people, ten of whom were tourists, in October 2004. Posing as friendly strangers, Djait and Samadi gave their victims drinks, coffee or lunch over a six-day period at various venues such as the Three Wise Monkeys bar on George Street, Sydney, The Shark Hotel on Liverpool Street, and the Pontoon Bar, The Opera Bar at Darling Harbour:

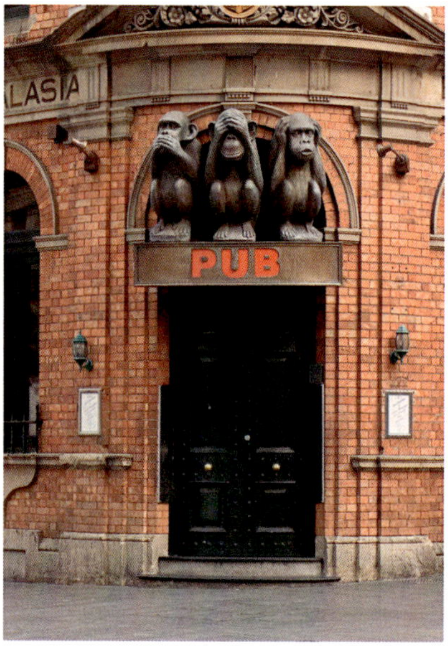


*Fig. 95: 'Three Wise Monkeys' bar, George Street, Sydney*

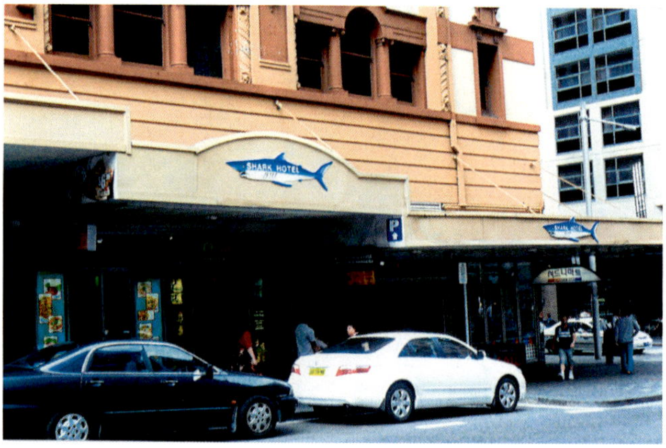


*Fig. 96: 'The Shark Hotel', Liverpool Street, Sydney*

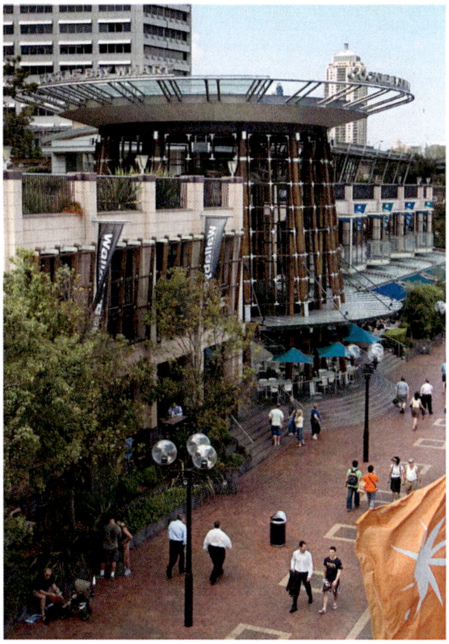

*Fig.97: 'Pontoon Bar', Darling Harbour, Sydney*

But their friendly charms masked an evil intent, as they proceeded to take cash, property and, in several instances, raped three and possibly four of their female victims while they were under the influence of the drug. The two men befriended their victims, bought drinks for them, then dropped the drug into the drinks apparently via a Tic-Tac dispenser. "[M]any awoke the next day with no memory of what happened and found their property had been stolen" or worse, had also been raped.

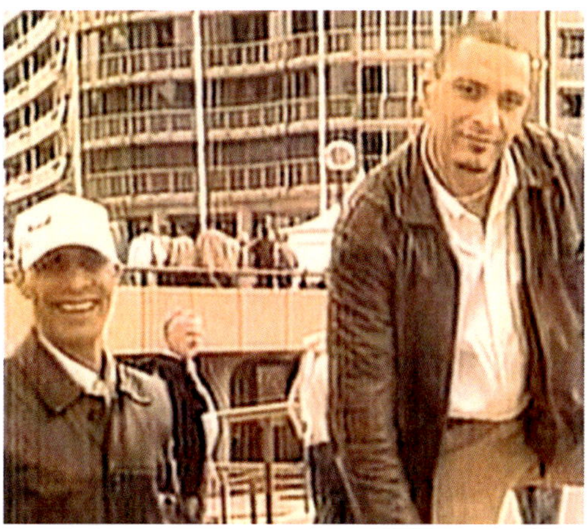

*Fig. 98: Adel Samadi ('Andy') and Chebli Djait ('Dylan')*

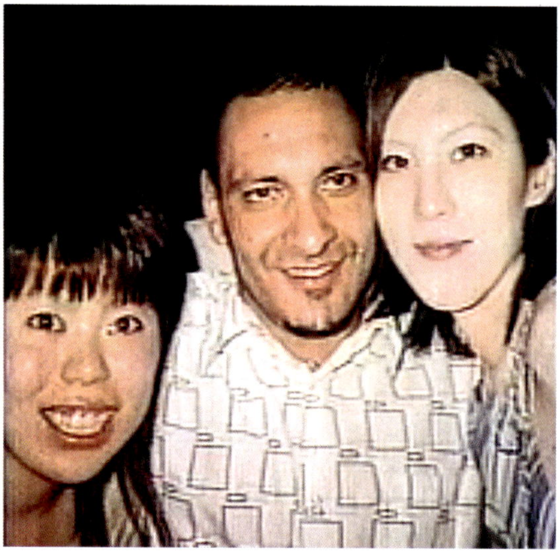

*Fig. 99: Chebli Djait in the company of two potential Asian victims*

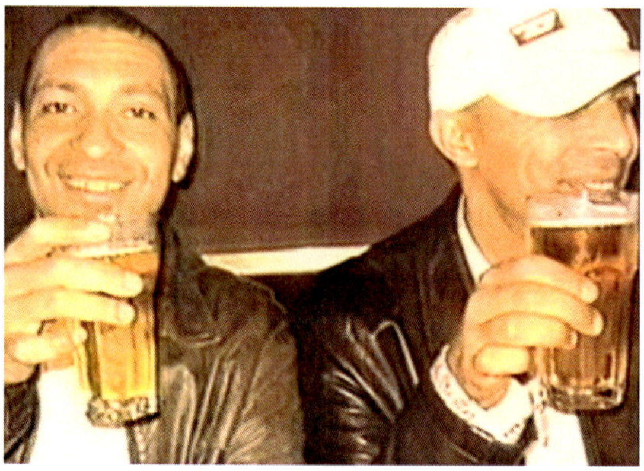

*Fig. 100: Chebli Djait ('Dylan') and Adel Samadi ('Andy') enjoying a beer during their nefarious activities*
*[Photographs: Courtesy Channel 7 News]*

After extensive enquiries by city detectives, spanning some weeks, they were soon onto the perpetrators: Chebli Djait of Peakhurst and Adel Samadi of Belmore alias 'Andy' and 'Dylan', after a number of complaints were reported to police. Djait was arrested in Kings Cross on October 19, 2004, and he was found in possession of a prescription for the drug, clonazepam. Samadi was arrested the following day and had two bottles of containing clonazepam in his possession. One bottle contained more than 85 tablets of Rivotril and a bottle of a white liquid containing clonazepam. These guys were clearly ready for further 'action' before being apprehended by police…

In all, the two villains had befriended ten women and two men at popular bars in inner Sydney before robbing them, and in a number of cases raping them. A rather nasty spree, and a terrible betrayal of trust to innocent tourists…

**Blood Analyses of Victims**

Blood samples were taken from some five victims – all tested positive for the drug: clonazepam, ranging from 0.015 to 0.030 milligrams per litre. To get this in perspective, the therapeutic level of this drug is 0.01-0.024 milligrams per litre. With one victim well outside this range. Two other victims only provided urine samples, in which clonazepam was also detected. It was obvious more than a therapeutic dosage had been administered to some of their victims, to ensure they were completely under the influence of the drug…

**Court**

I attended Sydney Central Court for the initial hearing, and gave evidence as to the levels of drug found in some of the victims' blood samples. As none of the victims were mentioned as suffering from epilepsy, then the levels of clonazepam found in their blood ranging from 0.015-0.030 mg/mL was "one and a half to three times above the lower end of the therapeutic concentration."

In other words, a good deal more than was necessary to achieve the outcome the villains sought…

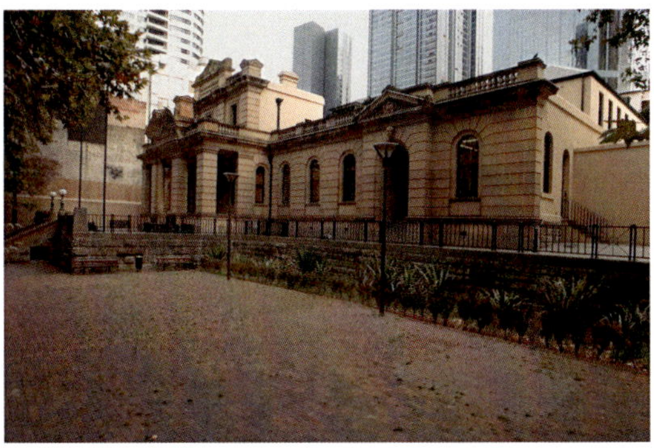

*Fig. 101: Sydney Central Court, Sydney, NSW.*

The Court heard that most of the victims were approached by 'Andy' and 'Dylan' while they drank in various groups at bars such as the Three Wise Monkeys on George Street, The Shark Hotel on Liverpool Street or Pontoon Bar and Opera Bar at Darling Harbour, Sydney. They then allegedly slipped the drug into their drinks and waited until their victims were incapacitated.

Three women were allegedly sexually assaulted while property including cash, credit cards, cameras and mobile phones were stolen from others…

A twenty-four-year-old Korean student described her harrowing ordeal after meeting with 'Andy' and 'Dylan' at the Shark Hotel on October 17, 2004. After the usual introductions, the pair 'shouted' [paid for] three rounds of drinks. The young lady went on to say, "I had a Midori and pineapple juice… while we talking I lost my memory, I don't remember leaving the hotel." She was apparently helped to her room before a number of sexual activities were carried out. She woke the following morning and recalls brief sections of the encounter:

"My eyes were open but I could not see properly. I couldn't think properly. I couldn't resist. He took off my underwear."

The Court then heard, "that she spent most of the day in a drugged sleep and during this time, was assaulted some three times" by 'Andy'.

Another victim, a twenty-two-year-old Japanese tourist, said she did not recall leaving the Three Wise Monkeys bar, but woke up the next morning in bed with a man she knew as 'Andy'.

Ms Susan Alexander, Head of Regulatory Affairs at Roche which markets the drug Rivotril, also gave evidence as to the effects of clonazepam. She said that:

"Clonazepam belongs to a family of drugs which also includes Rohypnol – notorious for its abuse by predatory drink-spikers."

Ms Alexander continued, "Rohypnol now contains a dye to warn of its presence in drinks, but clonazepam would not change colour or taste of the liquid… Unlike Rohypnol, prior to this case there had been no evidence that Rivotril was being used as a 'substance of abuse'…"

[Note: Unfortunately, I had several cases on file in which clonazepam had in fact been used in this manner on a number occasions in the past.]

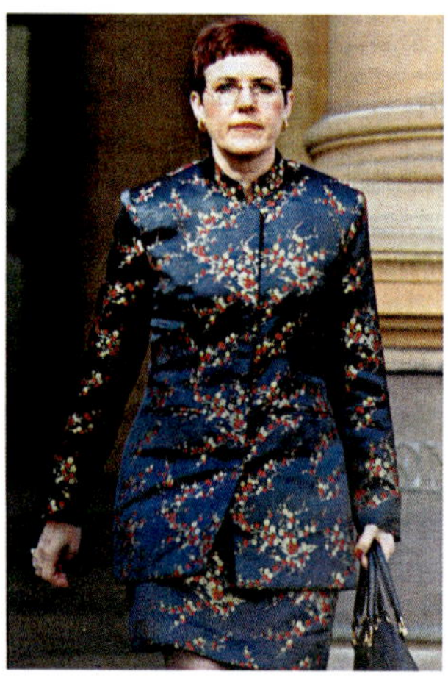

*Fig. 102: Ms. Susan Alexander after leaving Court –*
*Photograph courtesy of* The Daily Telegraph *July 28, 2005*

Clearly, witnesses had provided enough evidence against the pair for the matter to now go to District Court.

**A Lucky Escape - and Not So Lucky**

As the trial began in the Downing Centre District Court presided over by Judge Robyn Tupman, the jury was told the alleged attacks by 'Andy' and 'Dylan' in inner-Sydney bars bore a characteristic *modus operandi*:

"The two men befriended them, bought drinks for them, then dropped a drug in the drinks... many awoke the next day with no memory of what happened and found their property had been stolen," Crown Prosecutor Natalie Adams told the Court. She further added, "In two instances, women were sexually assaulted."

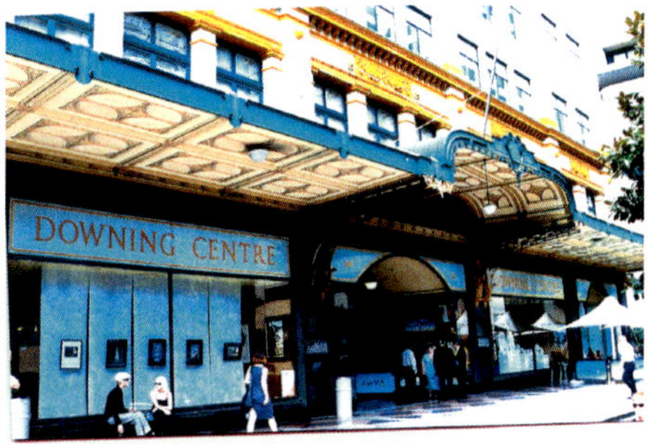


*Fig. 103: Downing Centre Court, Sydney*

Ms Adams said seven of the victims had blood tests the day after their experiences with Djiat and Samadi and all tested positive for clonazepam in their blood and two in their urine, despite none of them having ever taken the drug before or suffered from epilepsy.

The first alleged victim to give evidence was Ms Tracey Vo, who described feeling "hazy... and felt really, really, really drunk" and "I just wasn't seeing straight and from that point, parts of the evening black out", after she and a friend were given drinks by 'Andy' and 'Dylan'. She was able to get to the safety of a friend's hotel room before passing out.

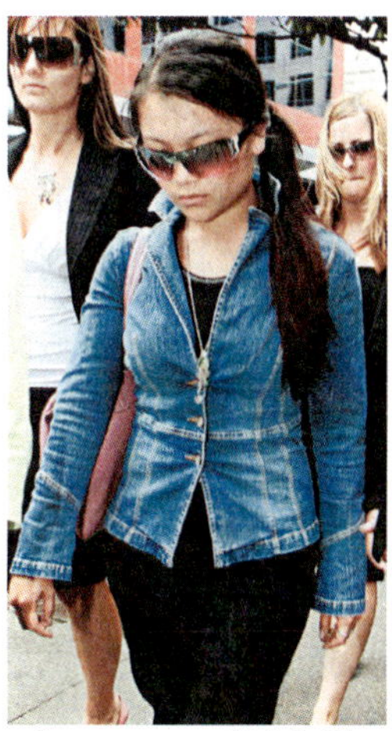

*Fig. 104: 'One that escaped' Ms Tracey Vo leaving*
*Photograph courtesy of* The Daily Telegraph *July 28, 2005*

Other victims were not quite so lucky…

Another victim, a male, invited the two villains home with him for a glass of wine, only to wake up the next day to discover the $17,000 worth of property had been stolen. DNA matching Samadi was found on a sock in the apartment and Djait's fingerprints were found on a door.

Another victim said she woke up on a mattress in Djait's unit fully clothed. However, she found that she was, "unable to move her head or body" being essentially 'paralysed'. The man she knew as 'Andy' (Djait) then allegedly removed her clothes and had sex with her.

Djait faced three charges of sexually assaulting a Korean tourist at his apartment and Samadi one charge of sexually assaulting a Swedish woman at a Kings Cross backpackers' hostel. Semen found on her sheets matched Samadi's DNA. Most of the victims were tourists, a number had property stolen and all suffered from memory loss – one of the characteristics of benzodiazepine ingestion.

In all there were twelve victims from the Djait and Samadi rampage, four were Japanese, two Korean, one Swiss, one Swedish, a person from Perth, a person from Adelaide and two from Sydney – the evil pair had indeed been very busy…

**The Outcome**

Adel Samadi and Chebli Djait were sentenced to fifteen years behind bars, with a non-parole period of twelve years, for drugging, robbing and raping, after an almost week-long drink-spiking spree at inner-Sydney bars. In sentencing the pair Judge Robyn Tupman said, "drink spiking is serious and potentially fatal. There should be a strong message of general deterrence sent by the sentence imposed here."

The Judge also found it, "disturbing that a doctor prescribed them the drug, Makram Girgis in a joint consultation and apparently did not monitor their treatment."

And further, "It was their ready access to this drug, in an apparently uncontrolled manner, which made their commission of these offences so much easier."

Dr Girgis said he did not recall a joint consultation, which would have been rather strange given the use of clonazepam. However, he later said to reporters, "The matter is in police hands and the medical board and the HCCC [Health Care Complaints Commission]… so I'm so terribly sorry but I can't give you the information."

**A 'Bit of Courtroom Drama'**

Djait's partner, Cheryl Khoury of Roselands, Sydney, had attended Court while he and his partner-in-crime, Samadi faced sentencing for their crimes.

Apparently, Khoury in the meantime had made about forty-six threatening phone calls to two of the female witnesses urging them not to testify along with threats, “In half an hour you’re going to be killed. You’re going to die. We are watching you from outside now.”

When one of the witnesses asked Khourr about the threats, Khoury replied, “Because you sent the two guys to jail and you’re going to court.” Furthermore, “If you think the Police are gunna save you, they can’t save you, believe me. You put somebody in jail, you gunna pay.”

These threats were levelled at two Japanese women who were among the twelve people who had their drinks spiked by Djait and his accomplice, Samadi. In another conversation, she apparently said, “You caused big trouble. I know where you live, I know where you work, I know everything about you.” The woman clearly had no idea what was going on and clearly sought revenge on whoever threatened ‘her man’ – right or wrong!

She was charged with two counts of threatening a person with intent to influence a witness.

As Khoury waited in the public gallery prior to sentencing for threatening witnesses, she collapsed dramatically to the floor, crying repeatedly, “I’m having an anxiety attack! Get me some tablets!”

She was helped from the floor by relatives and subsequently left the courtroom in tears. Was this an extraordinary bit of acting?

**A Prequel**

Just under two months later, Khoury appeared before NSW district court Judge Ronald Solomon and pleaded guilty to the two counts of threatening a person with intent to influence a witness.

Khoury’s psychiatrist, Dr Monier Younan gave evidence on her behalf stating, his “patient suffered from a complex psychiatric condition with a mixture of psychiatric disorders. These include obsessive compulsive disorder, chronic anxiety, post traumatic stress and depression.”

In consideration of Dr Younan’s evidence, Judge Solomon recognised that Khoury’s offences deserved a custodial sentence he said it would be “cruel and inhumane to send her to gaol” and further added, “If I send this offender to full-time custody I would be perpetrating a harsh and unnecessary punishment.”

He then handed down a twelve-month suspended gaol term for each offence. She was also placed on a two-year good behaviour bond. When handing down the sentence, Judge Solomon said, “It appears to me that out of a misplaced sense of duty and out of a strong love for Mr Djait that the defendant committed these offences.”

Khoury did not know just how lucky she had been. This offence carries a maximum penalty of ten years imprisonment! – and what of the victims she threatened? One wonders whether justice prevailed that day…

[At the time of writing, it appeared indeed that Dr Girgis was under investigation by the Police and the Health Care Complaints Commission. However, nothing appears to be done in regard to the controlling the prescribing of clonazepam as the scheduling has not been changed. Hopefully, this will soon occur as with flunitrazepam or Rohypnol.]

# 14
# Methadone Mothers

*"I didn't think the little bit that I gave him would've killed him."*
Methadone Mum

## Introduction

Methadone, also known as Physeptone and Dolophine, was first synthesised by German chemists during World War II as a morphine substitute. The drug is a powerful analgesic used to relieve moderate to severe pain from a variety of sources including, trauma, surgery, heart attack and burns. The drug has also been used to treat the pain in cases of terminal cancer where it eases the suffering and provides a feeling of euphoria and peace – very desirable outcomes for the terminally ill. Also, it is more reliable than morphine when given by mouth.

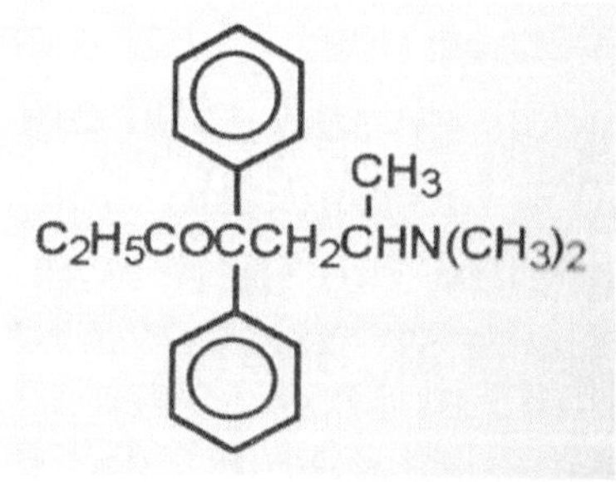


*Fig. 105: Chemical structure of methadone.*

However, unlike morphine, methadone produces a marked sedative effect and with repeated doses can result in a drug build-up. This is due to its rather long half-life of fifteen to fifty-five hours (average twenty-five hours, whereas morphine is only 2.5 hours) with resultant toxic effects. The drug has proven useful as a direct substitute for opiate (heroin) users to help them minimise drug usage before withdrawal symptoms develop, and has been used for some time for addicts to control their habit. Hence the use of the drug in various rehabilitation programs to wean heroin addicts off their habit. Since the inception of methadone maintenance clinics in the late 1960s, accidental poisoning (and in some cases, deliberate poisoning) of children with methadone has been reported in the literature and the news media:

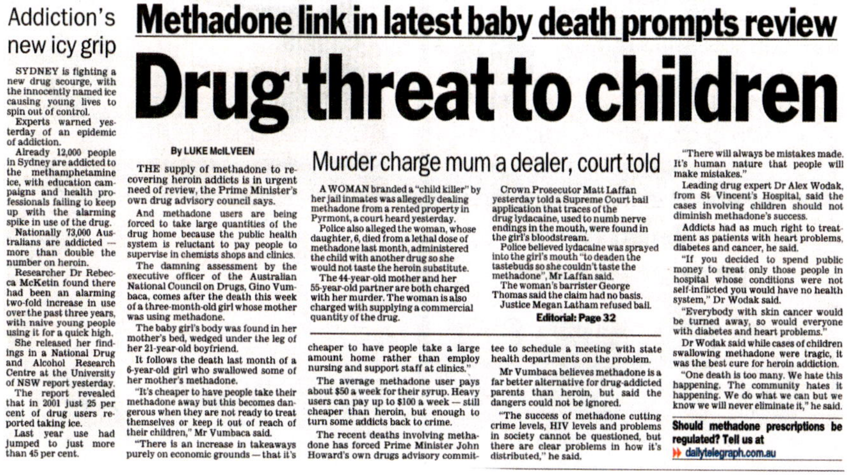

Addiction's new icy grip

SYDNEY is fighting a new drug scourge, with the innocently named ice causing young lives to spin out of control.

Experts warned yesterday of an epidemic of addiction.

Already 12,000 people in Sydney are addicted to the methamphetamine ice, with education campaigns and health professionals failing to keep up with the alarming spike in use of the drug.

Nationally 73,000 Australians are addicted — more than double the number on heroin.

Researcher Dr Rebecca McKetin found there had been an alarming two-fold increase in use over the past three years, with naive young people using it for a quick high.

She released her findings in a National Drug and Alcohol Research Centre at the University of NSW report yesterday.

The report revealed that in 2001 just 25 per cent of drug users reported taking ice.

Last year use had jumped to just more than 45 per cent.

Methadone link in latest baby death prompts review

Drug threat to children

By LUKE McILVEEN

THE supply of methadone to recovering heroin addicts is in urgent need of review, the Prime Minister's own drug advisory council says.

And methadone users are being forced to take large quantities of the drug home because the public health system is reluctant to pay people to supervise in chemists shops and clinics.

The damning assessment by the executive officer of the Australian National Council on Drugs, Gino Vumbaca, comes after the death this week of a three-month-old girl whose mother was using methadone.

The baby girl's body was found in her mother's bed, wedged under the leg of her 21-year-old boyfriend.

It follows the death last month of a 6-year-old girl who swallowed some of her mother's methadone.

"It's cheaper to have people take their methadone away but this becomes dangerous when they are not ready to treat themselves or keep it out of reach of their children," Mr Vumbaca said.

"There is an increase in takeaways purely on economic grounds — that it's cheaper to have people take a large amount home rather than employ nursing and support staff at clinics."

The average methadone user pays about $50 a week for their syrup. Heavy users can pay up to $100 a week — still cheaper than heroin, but enough to turn some addicts back to crime.

The recent deaths involving methadone has forced Prime Minister John Howard's own drugs advisory committee to schedule a meeting with state health departments on the problem.

Mr Vumbaca believes methadone is a far better alternative for drug-addicted parents than heroin, but said the dangers could not be ignored.

"The success of methadone cutting crime levels, HIV levels and problems in society cannot be questioned, but there are clear problems in how it's distributed," he said.

"There will always be mistakes made. It's human nature that people will make mistakes."

Leading drug expert Dr Alex Wodak, from St Vincent's Hospital, said the cases involving children should not diminish methadone's success.

Addicts had as much right to treatment as patients with heart problems, diabetes and cancer, he said.

"If you decided to spend public money to treat only those people in hospital whose conditions were not self-inflicted you would have no health system," Dr Wodak said.

"Everybody with skin cancer would be turned away, so would everyone with diabetes and heart problems."

Dr Wodak said while cases of children swallowing methadone were tragic, it was the best cure for heroin addiction.

"One death is too many. We hate this happening. The community hates it happening. We do what we can but we know we will never eliminate it," he said.

Should methadone prescriptions be regulated? Tell us at dailytelegraph.com.au

Murder charge mum a dealer, court told

A WOMAN branded a "child killer" by her jail inmates was allegedly dealing methadone from a rented property in Pyrmont, a court heard yesterday.

Police also alleged the woman, whose daughter, 6, died from a lethal dose of methadone last month, administered the child with another drug so she would not taste the heroin substitute.

The 44-year-old mother and her 55-year-old partner are both charged with her murder. The woman is also charged with supplying a commercial quantity of the drug.

Crown Prosecutor Matt Laffan yesterday told a Supreme Court bail application that traces of the drug lydacaine, used to numb nerve endings in the mouth, were found in the girl's bloodstream.

Police believed lydacaine was sprayed into the girl's mouth "to deaden the tastebuds so she couldn't taste the methadone", Mr Laffan said.

The woman's barrister George Thomas said the claim had no basis.

Justice Megan Latham refused bail.

Editorial: Page 32

*Fig. 106: "Drug Threat to Children"*
*[Source: 'Daily Telegraph']*

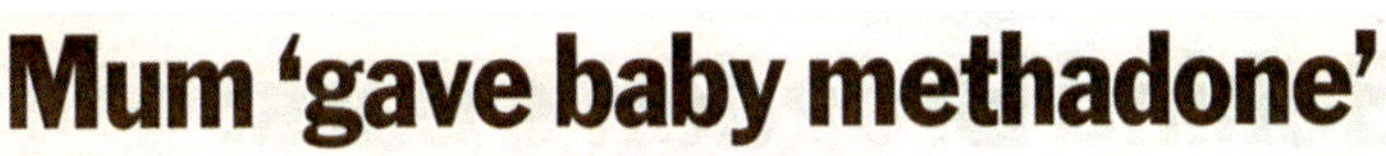

Mum 'gave baby methadone'

*Fig. 107: "Mum 'gave baby methadone'*
*[Courtesy 'Daily Telegraph']*

The toxic effects of the drug are more likely to occur in naive users before any tolerance has developed. For a relatively naïve user, the starting dose is initially 10-20 milligrams (mg) per day, rising to a maintenance range of 30-50 mg per day (maximum 80 mg/day), with an average range of 30-40 mg per day.

Aside from tablets, methadone is commonly supplied to addicts on a programme in the form of an orange flavoured syrup containing 5 mg/ml of the drug – which can be attractive to young children.

Methadone does not exert its full effects immediately after ingestion, so it is possible to take a large dose without any immediate perception by the user of a life-threatening intoxication. There is often a time gap of several hours between taking the drug and eventual collapse, allowing naïve users to think "the drug isn't working". So another dose is ingested, resulting in deep sedation and breathing difficulties, which steadily get worse depending upon how much was taken – with a possible fatal outcome. Unfortunately, 'methadone mums' (female heroin addicts undergoing therapy, with kids) have used the drug for its sedative effects on their youngsters for various reasons, as these three cases illustrate:

**Case 1. 'Teething Troubles'**

Baby Brent Partridge was apparently a healthy, happy eighteen-month-old boy who spent the last day of his life playing on the floor of his parent's unit. However, his playing area was like no other, empty methadone bottles and syringes were left scattered around the unit and young Brent was apparently allowed to play with the syringe barrels ".like a toy." The child was living in a world where both his parents – mum, Holly Davies and dad, Michael Partridge, and another couple Peter and Deanna Young, who were all heroin addicts – were attending a methadone clinic, supposedly to kick the habit. Holly apparently, supplemented her income through prostitution…

**A Busy Night**

It had been a busy night with one client after another coming into the brothel.

This mother had had a busy night – and profitable too. Holly and her friend, Deanna, had been out all night, working as prostitutes, before returning to their shared unit in the wee small hours of the morning at about five a.m., 14 November, 1995.

"Come on, I'm exhausted, let's go home…"

**A Drugged Child**

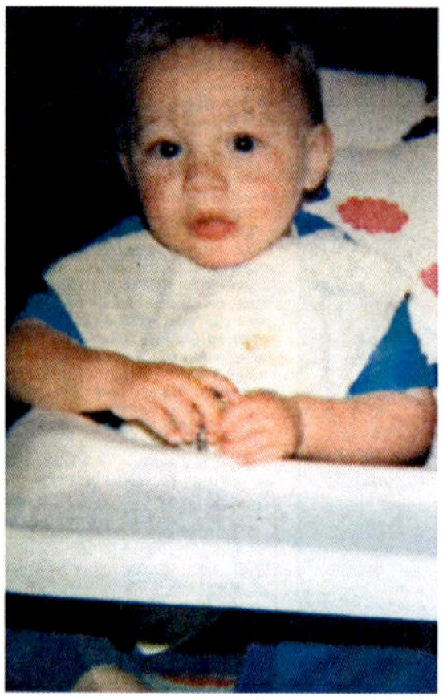

*Fig. 108: Baby Brent Partridge in happier days.*
*[Courtesy* The Daily Telegraph *February 5, 2003, p. 17].*

Holly's baby boy of eighteen months was experiencing the arrival of his first teeth, and this was causing him some discomfort, aside from a viral infection. Maybe some methadone would help… The baby boy, Brent, was restless, and Holly apparently gave him "a tiny little bit" of methadone to soothe his teething pains – and may well have taken some herself, as both Mum and her baby then fell asleep in the lounge chair. The baby lay stomach down on his mother's lap in the lounge chair. Hours passed, and Holly eventually awoke at one p.m. and placed the child on a lounge chair, where he apparently appeared to be still asleep. Unfortunately, he wasn't. He was in a deep drug-induced coma – and his life had ebbed away. The father of the child, Michael Partridge went to place him into his cot in the bedroom at about three p.m., when he noticed that he was not moving – and had turned blue in complexion. This was not good, and an ambulance was called, along with the Police, who arrived a short time later. The residence was in a state of disarray and the bedroom very untidy, with dirty clothes and other items strewn throughout the floor, cot and bed of the residence. The ambulance arrived at about three twenty p.m., and found that the child had been dead for some hours. It was later ascertained that baby Brent Partridge had been dead for up to six hours before Holly realised anything was wrong…

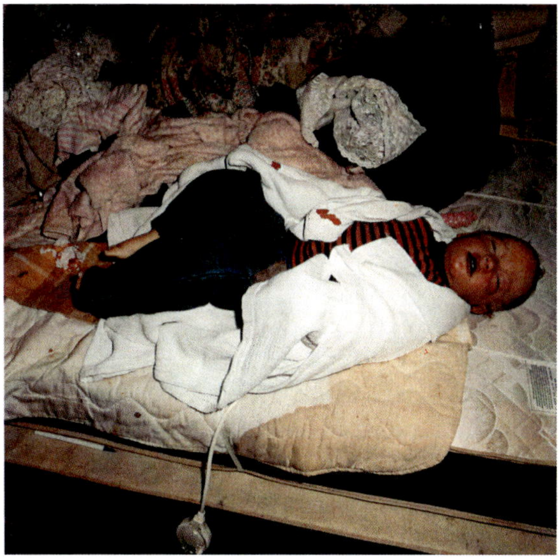

*Fig. 109: The child's body as he was found in the unit.*

**Blood Levels Found**

A blood sample taken from the deceased child at the post mortem was found to contain methadone 0.5 milligrams per litre. A high level even for an adult, let alone a toddler. The child's liver was found to contain 0.71 milligram per kilogram and the stomach contents (weighing about 27 grams) were found to contain 22 mg/kg of methadone (or about 0.6 mg). The level of methadone found in the toddler's blood was more than enough to result in the death of a child of this age.

**NSW HEALTH**
DEPARTMENT
DIVISION OF ANALYTICAL LABORATORIES

Joseph street, Lidcombe
Postal Address:
P.O. Box 162
Lidcombe, N.S.W. 2141

Reference: PARTRIDGE, Brent
Register Number: T952255

Telephone: (02) 646 0222
Facsimile: (02) 646 0333

I,

1.

2. The following described items, bearing the name PARTRIDGE, were received:

| ITEM | SECURITY DESCRIPTION | AMOUNT (approx.) |
|---|---|---|
| LIVER | sealed | 57 g |
| STOMACH | sealed | 27 g |
| BLOOD (preserved) | sealed | 10 mL |
| URINE | sealed | 5 mL |
| BILE | sealed | 1 mL |
| VITREOUS HUMOR | sealed | 1mL |

on 16/11/95 from MONTGOMERY , IOFM

3. The items have been examined with the following results:

Screening tests:
Comprehensive screening tests for drugs and other common poisons were performed.

Quantitative procedure results:

| | |
|---|---|
| BLOOD ALCOHOL: nil | |
| BLOOD (preserved) | Methadone: 0.50mg/L |
| LIVER | Methadone: 0.71mg/kg |
| STOMACH | Methadone: 22mg/kg |
| VITREOUS HUMOR | Alcohol: Not detected |

-9 FEB 1996

PATHOLOGIST:

Forwarded for your information coroner
GLEBE

(signature of analyst)

*Fig. 110: Analyst's Report – re: Brent Partridge.*

## Coroner's Court

There the matter lay, until it was taken to Glebe Coroner's Court in February, 2003, to try to answer the questions surrounding baby Brent's tragic death. In particular, how did the deadly drug get into his body? There initially appeared to be two likely scenarios, either one or both parents administered it in an effort to sedate him or, somehow, the toddler found some methadone syrup in a container lying on the floor. 'Take away' methadone is usually provided as an orange-flavoured syrup containing 5 milligrams per millilitre of the drug.

I estimated that for an infant weighing 18 kilograms, a minimum dosage of 24 to 28 milligrams (or 5-6 mls or about a teaspoon) would have had to been taken to achieve the methadone blood level found. Could the infant taken the drug himself? It seemed unlikely in my view, however…

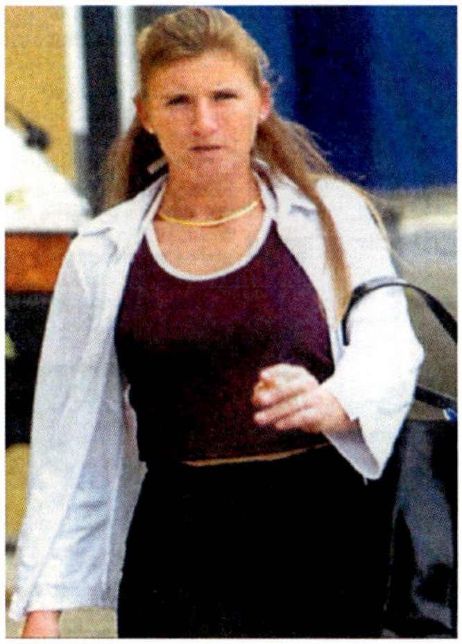

*Fig. 111: Brent's mother, Holly Davies at the Coroner's Court. [Courtesy* The Daily Telegraph *February 6, 2003 p.21]*

**Supreme Court**

Another two years had passed. In February, 2005 the parents of toddler Brent Partridge, who had some years earlier died from a methadone overdose, stood trial in the New South Wales Supreme Court, at Taylor Square, Darlinghurst charged with manslaughter. What was happening in the meantime?

In an unusual turn of events, Holly Davies and Michael Partridge stood trial before a judge alone, namely Justice David Kirby, with no jury being present.

The Crown Prosecutor, Richard Herps, in making his opening remarks, told the Court that both the accused were on a methadone program at the time of the toddler's death and had taken some of the drug that morning. He further told the Court that the prosecution will allege that the child was either given the methadone as a sedative or the child consumed the drug himself while his parents were asleep.

The defence solicitor, Phil Gibson took the latter position. He was aided by the fact that a 1997 report describing the child's death through methadone intoxication had sat in the Coroner's Court for years, while recordings, Police notes and methadone exhibits had been destroyed. These matters were raised by his Honour. Unfortunately, I hadn't requested that the boy's hair be tested for methadone. If the drug was present, this would have been very useful information to determine whether the methadone ingestion was a 'one-off' or a chronic ingestion which would have indicated a neglect of the child.

Ms Davies apparently confessed to her brother, Michael Ford that several weeks after Brent Partridges's death that she deliberately gave him methadone. According to a statement Mr Ford made to police, the conversation apparently went like this: "I want to talk to you about Brent."

"What do you want to tell me?" he asked.

"He must have licked that methadone off a spoon," she replied.

"We are talking about an eighteen-month-old baby darling, to my mind that would be impossible. Did you give it to him?"

Sobbing, Holly then said to her brother, "I didn't think the little bit that I gave him would've killed him. I just wanted to ease the pain that he was in."

Well, that certainly was achieved. More importantly, Mr Ford admitted that his sister was intoxicated at the time of the confession.

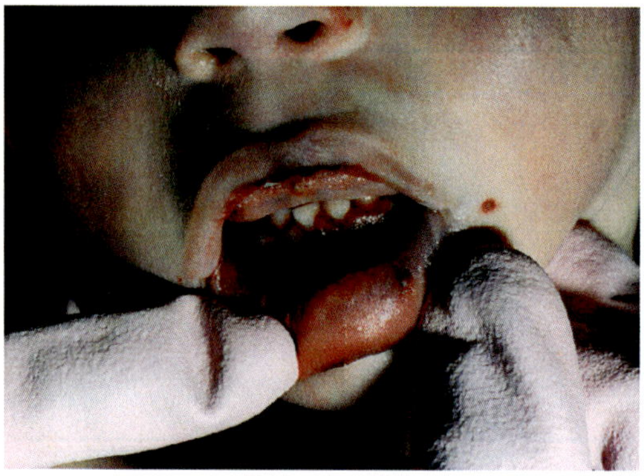

*Fig. 112: Close up of baby Brent Partridge showing teething problems.*

The prosecution said Mr Ford's account supported the evidence given by Kathryn Adams, who has a daughter with one of Holly Davies' brothers, said that she had given methadone to toddler Brent for teething pain. This seemed to confirm the methadone for teething problems scenario.

Unfortunately, Mr Ford had since died from cancer and so could not be cross-examined on this issue.

**The Outcome**

Justice Kirby found that the prosecution failed to produce enough evidence that methadone was deliberately given to the child or that there was criminal negligence by Davies or her de facto husband, Partridge. Therefore, there was insufficient evidence for a conviction over the death of Brent Partridge – and so they were cleared over the child's methadone death.

Outside the Court, Davies' solicitor Phil Gibson, said his client was relieved. – Hardly surprising, since she had admitted much earlier she had given him "a tiny little bit". My guess is that this was a teaspoon or more, maybe a small amount to an addict, but a fatal amount for a toddler.

As Ms Davies' solicitor said, "It is still a tragedy, and Holly has to live with the tragedy of Brent's death every day." And yes, and he would have been approaching his eighteenth birthday (at the time of writing, 2013), and if this tragedy had not occurred, had his whole life ahead of him but for "a tiny bit [of methadone]" to ease teething pain.

## Case 2. 'Sleepless in Bermagui'

### Introduction

Bermagui is a relaxed, attractive fishing and surfing village on the Far South Coast of New South Wales. Zane Grey placed Bermagui on the global calendar and established the birthplace of game fishing for black marline and yellow fin tuna in the 1930s, which continues today.

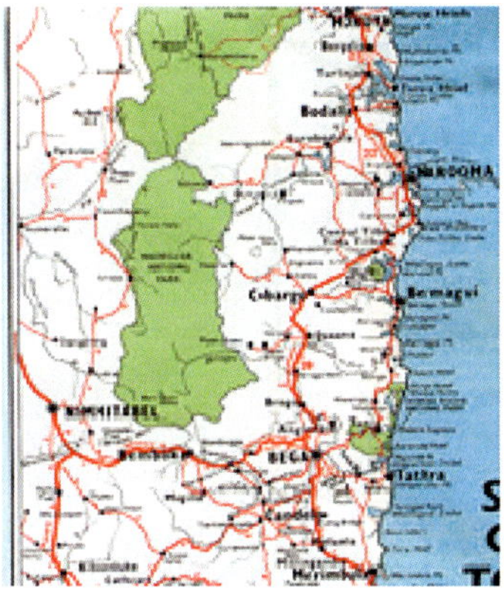

Fig. 113.

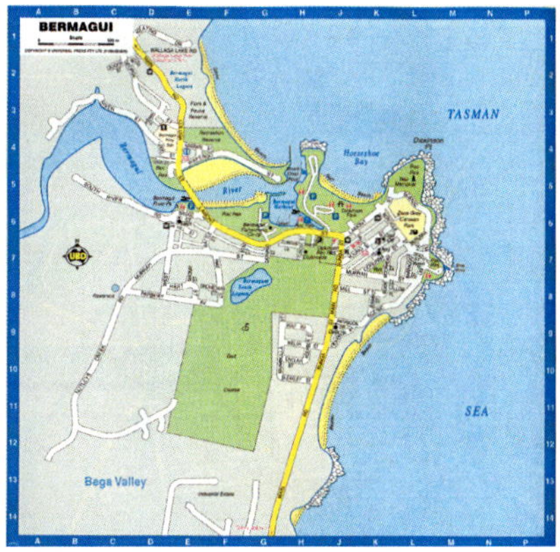


Fig. 114

*Figs. 113, 114: Maps of Bermagui, on the Sapphire Coast.*
*[Courtesy NSW Travel Bureau]*

It is a wonderful tourist destination on the Sapphire Coast and not a place you would not expect problems that this case unfolded…

### Another Drugged Child

Young Tyson Gray-McGregor was a happy, healthy four-year-old boy who lived with his mother, Naomi Gray and his nine-year-old sister, Kelli, in Bermagui.

Naomi, being a single mum found things difficult and found friendship in the form of Alan Thornton, who was from another South Coast town of Moruya.

The friendship developed, and Alan was invited to stay the night at Naomi's home on the 17 January, 2005. Unfortunately, as things turned out, Alan Thornton was on a local methadone program for opiate (heroin) dependency problems. At that time his daily dosage was 26 millilitres of methadone syrup supplied at a strength of 5 milligrams per millilitre, giving an effective daily dose of 130 milligrams of methadone. A fairly strong dosage, indicating he was in the early stage of his methadone program. But, the kids were excited, 'Uncle Alan is staying over!' and so could not sleep.

Tyson in particular was more restless and his mother and 'Uncle' Alan were having difficulty in getting him to settle and go to sleep. This apparently posed some problems, as both children were sleeping in the same bedroom. At about ten thirty p.m. Tyson was apparently still wide awake and more 'drastic measures' were no doubt discussed, including giving him some methadone syrup in a drink to get him to go to sleep…

As it had been a late night, both Naomi Gray and Alan Thornton had slept in until about nine forty-five a.m. Naomi awoke, and not hearing the children playing, which she thought unusual, she went into the children's bedroom. She saw both children still lying in their respective beds and thought they were both still asleep. She then went over to check Tyson and saw he was blue around the lips and cold to touch. He was apparently dead, and had been dead for some hours as post mortem lividity and rigor mortis had already set in. She screamed out to her boyfriend, Alan Thornton and he came running into the room. Attempts at CPR (cardiac pulmonary resuscitation) were fruitless and the Police and an ambulance were called. Later, Tyson's little body was collected and taken for a post mortem to determine the cause of his death.

About two weeks later, Alan Thornton admitted to a witness before the child's funeral that he put some methadone in a cordial given to Tyson to make him settle, and that he "must have put in too much." The addition of the methadone to the child's drink was done with the knowledge and consent of his mother…

**Blood Levels Found**

A blood sample taken from the deceased child at the post mortem was found to contain methadone 0.3 milligrams per litre. This level was again more than enough to result in the death of a child of this age. In addition, 1.3 milligrams of methadone was found in his bile – indicating some time had elapsed prior to his death

**A Suicide Attempt – an Admission of Guilt?**

It would appear that Alan Thornton's admission to a witness before the child's funeral, that he put some methadone in a cordial given to Tyson to make him settle, appeared to have preyed on his mind. In addition, this was done with the knowledge and consent of Tyson's mother. Both parties were apparently remorseful, and due to a drug overdose were unable to attend Tyson's funeral. A deliberate overdose of methadone? In any case, both parties fortunately recovered in hospital and were able to attend court.

**Court – and Drug Levels**

The drug was apparently given to the child to 'help make him sleep' and it certainly achieved that – with a fatal outcome. In opposing bail, police told the court they had evidence that Thornton had given Tyson methadone in a cordial drink because "he would not settle [sleep] for the night." Magistrate David

Helipern refused Thornton bail, but released Gray (Tyson's mother) on the condition she reported to police at Bermagui three times a week. I attended the court at Bega and advised legal council in the matter. The level of methadone that was present in his blood was more than sufficient to result in the death of the child. It appeared that a minimum of just over half a teaspoon of methadone syrup had been administered to the child, assuming the original mixture was at the usual concentration of methadone 5 milligrams per millilitre. Given the level of the drug was present in the child's bile, it is likely more of the drug had been given to 'settle him'.

## The Outcome

Tyson's mother Naomi Gray (thirty-two) received a twenty-one month suspended gaol sentence when she was sentenced before Justice McLoughlin in Bega Court on 8 March, 2007. The suspension was conditional that she entered a good behaviour bond and be under the directions of her parole officer at all times for the duration of the bond. Ms Gray's partner at the time of young Tyson's death, Alan Thornton, had previously pleaded guilty to manslaughter in connection with the boy's death and received a six-year sentence with a non-parole period of four years.

## Case 3. 'Bye Bye Baby'

## Feeding Time

It was a cool early morning at about five a.m. on 23 August 2006 when Sheila Kelly (not her real name) was apparently breastfeeding her three-week-old baby daughter, Michelle Kelly (not her real name) in the rear room of their house. A purely natural thing to do with a newborn baby. Unfortunately, this morning was going to be very different, as the baby began to choke. She turned blue and stopped breathing for no apparent reason. Sheila screamed, "My baby, my baby!" and woke her partner, Lee Townsend (not his real name) who was sleeping in the lounge room. Upon hearing her screams, Lee ran to the rear room where had been Sheila feeding their child.

## Emergency

He noticed a wet patch around the baby's head and some blood coming from the child's nose. This was odd – and very disturbing, and why after just breast feeding? The 000 number was promptly called for an ambulance to attend. The ambulance arrived a short time later and attempted to resuscitate the baby. At about five forty a.m. ambulance officers conveyed the baby and her mother to Campbelltown Hospital. At five forty-four a.m. the ambulance arrived at the hospital and handed the baby to hospital staff. Intensive efforts were made by hospital staff to resuscitate the baby, but were unsuccessful. At five fifty-six a.m. baby Michelle was declared deceased by a doctor at Campbelltown Hospital.

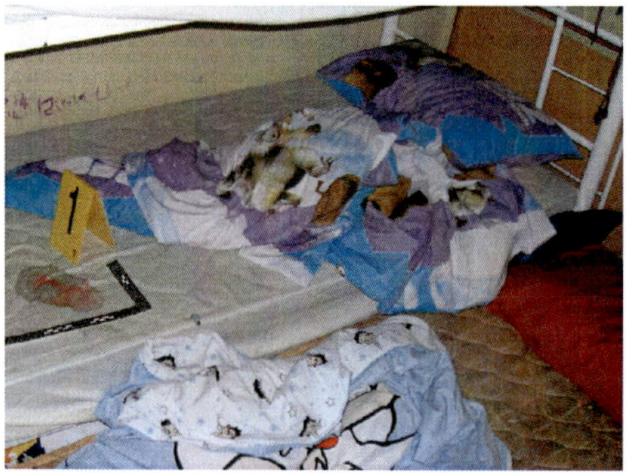

*Fig. 115: The stained bed linen*

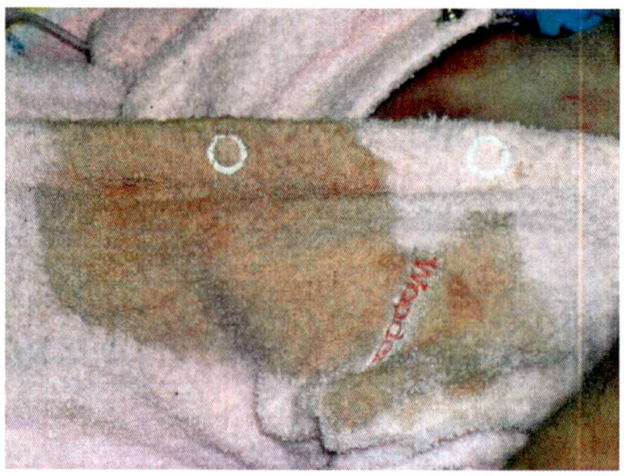

*Fig. 116: Close-up of the stained bed linen*

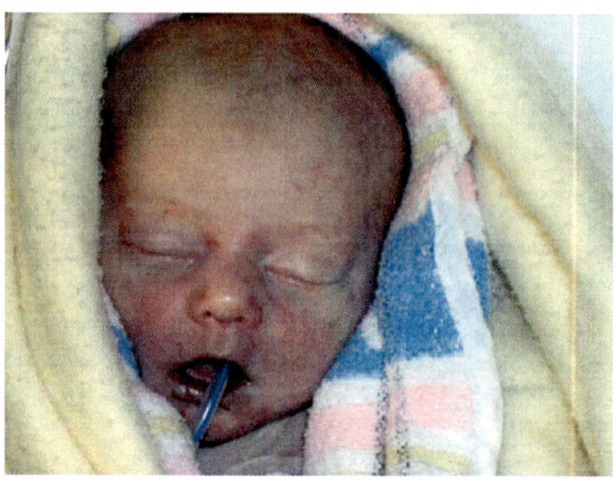

*Fig. 117: Baby Michelle.*

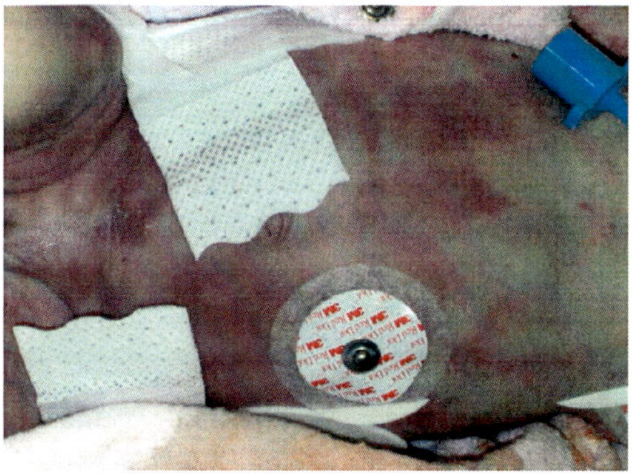

*Fig. 118: With resuscitation attempts on her little body [Photos: Campbelltown Crime Scene, NSW Police Force]*

However, Sheila apparently could not accept that her baby daughter was dead.

When police officers arrived at Campbelltown Hospital they found her sitting in a chair holding the deceased baby in her left arm. Sheila had her head resting on a bed and was crying. Her deceased baby was wrapped in a yellow blanket and a tube was still in her mouth from earlier resuscitation attempts. She remained sitting, holding the baby and was continually crying and talking to the dead baby asking her to wake up "Wake up baby, wake up..!" Eventually, Sheila stood up and placed her deceased baby in a cot beside her and walked out of the room.

At twelve p.m. a Government contractor arrived and removed the baby's body which was then conveyed to the Westmead Hospital Forensic Medicine section.

**Blood Levels Found**

A blood sample taken from the deceased child at the post mortem was found to contain methadone 0.1 milligrams per litre. This level was again more than enough to result in the death of a child of this age. In addition, 0.4 milligrams per kilogram of methadone was found in her liver – indicating some time had elapsed prior to her death. Methadone was also detected in her stomach contents. Obviously, the baby had taken the drug orally…

**Yet Another Drugged Child**

The therapeutic range for methadone in adults is given as 0.05 – 1.0 mg/L. However, death may occur at low blood levels and the level detected in baby Michaela's blood was 0.1 milligrams per litre – given her age more than enough to seriously depress her central nervous system to the extent of causing her death. The risks of methadone to children and naïve users have been well documented, but little action appears to have been taken over the years to reduce these dreadful casualties. Little baby Kelly appeared to be yet another casualty, and the level appeared far too high to be a carry over from breast milk….

## The Outcome

The matter eventually went before the Coroner at Westmead, who found that there was insufficient evidence that methadone was deliberately given to the child or that there was criminal negligence by Ms Kelly. Astonishingly, an interstate expert suggested the methadone came from the mother's milk! An observation that is *not supported by the literature.* After much legal argument the Coroner returned an 'open finding' as the manner in which the baby had ingested the methadone could not be determined with any degree of certainty.

This was yet another case where another beautiful child was lost to methadone intoxication.

## Case 4. A young girl and a bottle of 'Biodone'

A six-year-old female was found deceased at the foot of her mother's bed. The household consisted of the six-year-old, her mother, her mother's de-facto husband and his two children.

The mother stated that on the Friday, two days prior to death, her six-year-old daughter had flu-like symptoms and had vomited on a number of occasions. The mother gave her some 'Dimetapp' (brompheniramine and phenylephrine) and Dymadon (paracetamol).

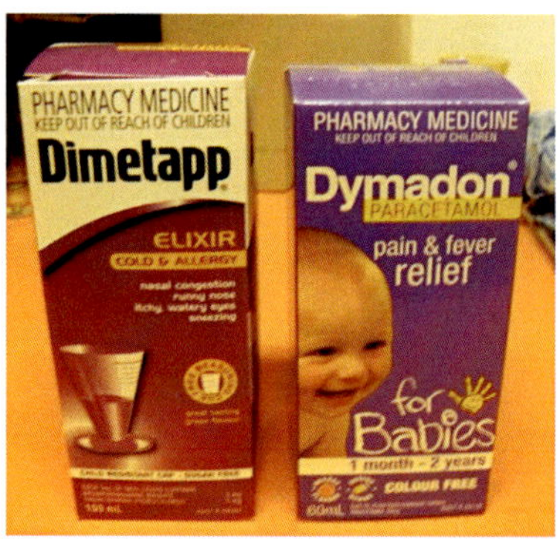


*Fig. 119: Typical Dimetapp and Dymadon preparations.*

The following day (Saturday), she was given some more Dimetapp and fell asleep. When she woke she vomited again. Around one thirty a.m. on Sunday, the child was asleep in her mother's bed, she was woken and taken to her own bed.

However around three a.m., the six-year-old asked her mother for some water and more Dimetapp. According to her mother she was very alert. The child then returned to her bed. Around seven a.m. on Sunday, the mother woke to find her daughter asleep at the foot of her bed and the mother said she was sleeping and breathing normally. At nine a.m. the de facto partner checked on the child and found she had no movement and was not breathing.

An ambulance was called and a doctor also attended and found the child was cyanosed, cold, had no pulse and was in asystole (no cardiac activity).

### The Mother

The mother stated she had been on methadone for about twelve years and she picked up take-away doses of methadone (35 mg) from her pharmacy. It was supplied in small brown bottles with a white cap under the trade name, Biodone.

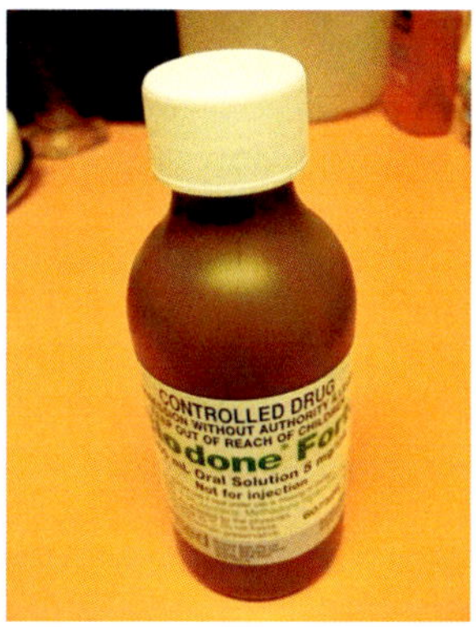


*Fig. 120: A typical Biodone syrup preparation.*

She allegedly had her prescriptions faxed to her by her doctor, which appeared very unusual. In the meantime, investigating police officers found some twenty-eight bottles of various sizes containing methadone in the house, including four 500 ml bottles of Biodone (methadone syrup) some with the tamper-proof manufacturer's seal still intact, two full 250 ml bottles and various smaller bottles. A total over three litres! The mother's explanation was she was "storing a bit" because she was on a pension!

(Note: Methadone would never be dispensed to a patient in commercial quantities in Australia).

Some syringes were also found in the house containing traces of methadone.

An interesting finding was a small brown, unlabelled bottle with a white pump cap which was subsequently found to contain lignocaine. The significance of this find would be apparent later in the investigation, as ambulance officers who attended to the deceased child did not administer this drug. Lignocaine, aside from being a local anaesthetic, is used to treat cardiac arrhythmias.

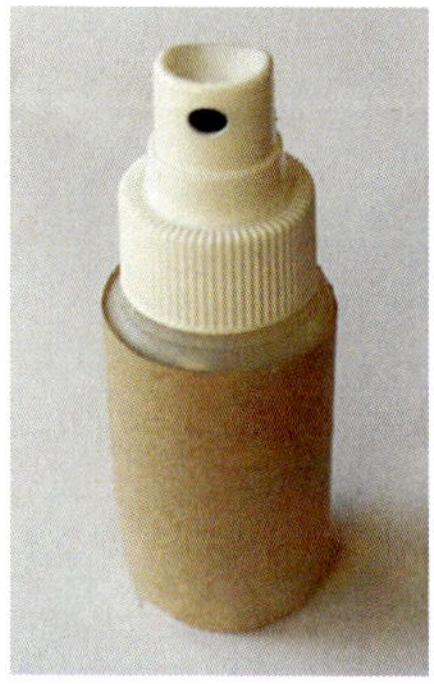

*Fig. 121: The lignocaine spray bottle.*

**The Toxicology Results.**

The six-year-old deceased girl was found to have a femoral blood concentration of methadone of 0.7 mg/L and lignocaine <0.1 mg/L. The stomach contents also indicated the presence of methadone (no level indicated), as did the liver (1.5 mg/kg). Later the deceased's hair sample was analysed and methadone was found to be present in each of seventeen two-centimetre segments of hair.

When reinterviewed the mother of the child indicated the small brown bottle with the white pump cap contained lignocaine which she used because the Biodone had a very unpleasant taste. The lignocaine spray was apparently used to 'deaden'(anaesthetise) the taste buds of the tongue!

**The Stepchildren**.

Whilst the Police were investigating the "suspicious" death of the six-year-old, the mother administered some Dimetapp to the two stepchildren. The older twelve-year-old later told the Police the mother usually gave them Dimetapp via a syringe. On this occasion (after the death of the six-year-old) when she was given the Dimetapp, it did not taste like Dimetapp. Both she had her younger sibling vomited after being given the medication and were later taken to hospital suffering from effects of methadone. They were both found to have methadone in their blood (< 0.1 mg/L). Was this a clever cover-up?

The mother then claimed she realised she must have given the same Dimetapp to her daughter and she realised it was Biodone in the bottle.

**The De-facto Partner**.

The de-facto partner did not use methadone but he was allegedly a user of prescribed dexamphetamine. He stated to police officers the mother put methadone in various bottles and had them in various places around the house.

## The Case for the Prosecution

It was alleged the mother had administered the deceased child some methadone, allegedly contained in a Dimetapp bottle and it was alleged the lignocaine was given to the child so that she would not react to the bitter taste of the drug (real Dimetapp has a very pleasant sweet taste which most children like).

The jury of eight women and four men were told the deceased girl had methadone in all segments of her hair which to an expert in hair analysis had indicated long term administration of methadone. Also, she had a fatal level of methadone in her blood. However, contrary to earlier evidence, at the trial, the hair expert suggested the findings in the hair may have resulted from vomit on the hair or close contact with the sweat from the mother's skin when she slept in her mother's bed.

(Note: The hair samples are washed with solvents before being subject to analysis.)

The de-facto partner, contrary to his earlier statement to the Police, stated he put the methadone into the Dimetapp box without the mother's knowledge.

The jury found the mother not guilty of manslaughter and not guilty of supplying a prohibited drug!

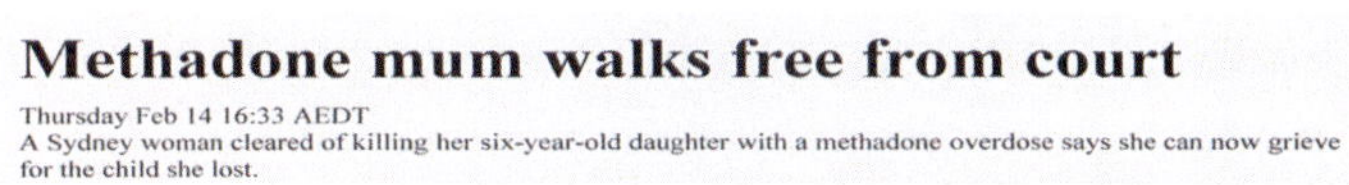

**Methadone mum walks free from court**

Thursday Feb 14 16:33 AEDT

A Sydney woman cleared of killing her six-year-old daughter with a methadone overdose says she can now grieve for the child she lost.

*Fig. 122: "Methadone mum walks free from court."*

**What the Jury was not told.**

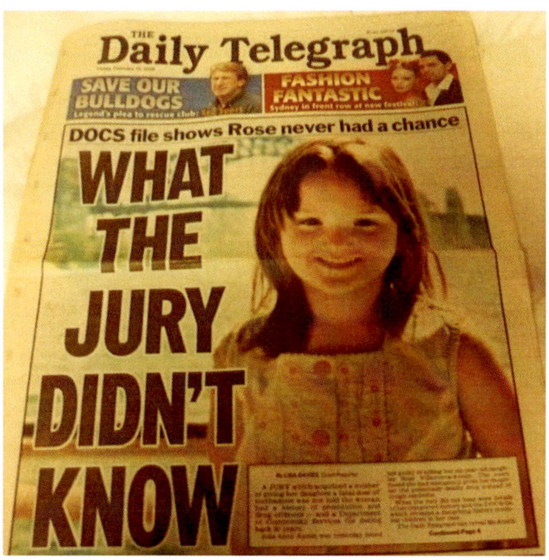


*Fig.123*: The Daily Telegraph *headlines, 'What the jury was not told'*

The mother had a history of prostitution and drug offences dating back twenty years and had a history with the Department of Community Services in relation to neglect of children in her care, including one child being admitted to hospital in an intoxicated state.

The natural father of the deceased child indicated he would sue the de-facto partner for the administration of methadone to his child and he also indicated he wanted an enquiry into the evidence given in relation to the hair analysis and the contradictory evidence of the expert.

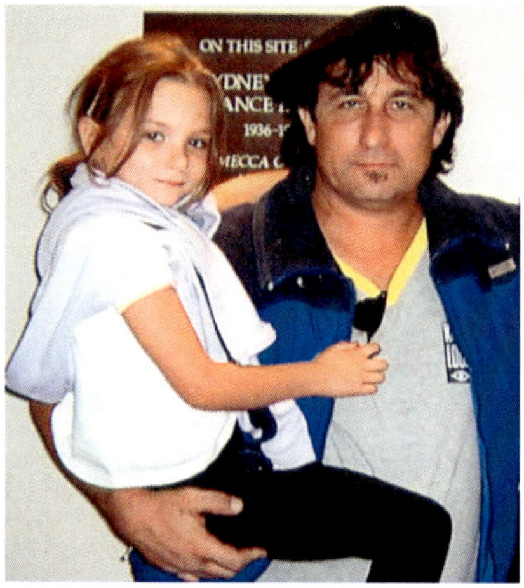


*Fig. 124*: *Father and daughter in happier times.*
*Courtesy:* The Daily Telegraph

**Conclusion**

Unfortunately, these cases are typical of the many encountered over the years, and illustrate the danger associated with takeaway methadone preparations particularly, for small children of parents undergoing treatment. The delay in seeking help in the majority of the cases appeared to be related to the parents' total unawareness of the danger inherent in methadone for their child until drowsiness and decreased respiration became quite apparent. Therefore, it is essential that strict legislative safety measures be implemented to eliminate this safety hazard for children of persons on a methadone maintenance program. One wonders how many more children will die from this drug before effective controls are put into practise.

# 15
# The Case of the One-Armed Would-be Rapist

*"First you take a drink, then the drink takes a drink, then the drink takes you."*
F. Scott Fitzgerald

## Introduction

Alcohol is the drug most commonly associated with sexual assault cases mainly due to its easy availability. It is rapidly absorbed into the bloodstream after ingestion and distributes through the entire body, including more importantly, the central nervous system where its depressant effects are most profound. In drug-facilitated sexual assault cases, the victims quite often consume the alcohol voluntarily, particularly when the perpetrator provides the alcoholic beverage in copious quantities to the potential victim. Alcohol decreases inhibitions, impairs perception and may cause loss of consciousness and/or amnesia, especially when other CNS drugs such as diazepam, for example, are used. This case was illustrative, with a surprising outcome…

## An Evening Out

It was a cool evening of 12 July when Sandra Clooney met up with Ken Grose (not their real names) a date for a social drink or drinks at the Five Dock Hotel. He was a fellow who had a hard life having lost an arm through an industrial accident, and was keen to get back on the social scene. Throughout the night Ken bought Sandra a number of drinks ranging from 'VB's ("Victoria Bitter" beers) to Sambuca drinks. Ms Clooney was clearly starting to be affected by the alcohol – big time, and was starting to become quite light-headed.

"Gosh, I feel pissed Ken."

Mr Grose realised things were starting to look promising – a sure thing?

He then goes to the bar and orders further drinks saying to the bar staff, "I'm going to get a root [have sex] tonight." He was a subtle romantic!

## Home to Bed?

Meanwhile, the further drinks were probably unnecessary, given what Ken Grose had in mind. By this time, Sandra was well 'under the weather' [very intoxicated] and quite incapable of getting herself home – the alcohol and other drug/s 'on board' ensured she was well and truly 'out to it'. Unfortunately, Sandra wasn't headed for home to sleep off her drink and what else was in her blood. She started to doze off. Slumped in Ken Grose's vehicle, she was soon in a deep sleep. Home to bed to sleep it off? No, other manoeuvres were afoot and Ken had other ideas…

Sandra was by now 'well out to it' and Ken Grose was also affected by alcohol. He stopped the motor vehicle and decided to carry out his fantasies. He opened the door and dragged Sandra out, both of them spilling into the gutter alongside the roadway. Time for some 'fun', he undid Sandra's jeans and pulled them down along with her panties, and unzipped the fly of his trousers…

**Sprung, 'Grose' by name Gross by Nature!**

Meanwhile a police officer, at a nearby Western Suburbs Soccer Club regarding another matter, was distracted by a male and female lying in the roadside gutter. The police officer called the manager and doorman of the Club to accompany him to the pair, where they see Sandra lying face down on the roadway with her jeans and panties down to her knees. Grose was observed lying on top of her whilst moving his pelvis up and down over her exposed bottom.

'Hey, what's going on here?' the officer asked.

When Grose was discovered, he stood up and revealed that his fly of his trousers was undone. Sandra was still unconscious. It was a very compromising situation to say the least. Sandra was taken to hospital and Grose was taken back to the police station and charged with Attempt Sexual Assault.

Meanwhile, Sandra regained consciousness at the hospital and was unaware of what happened to her. 'Where am I..? How did I get here..?' She was subjected to testing involving a Sexual Assault Investigation Kit (SAIK) where blood and urine samples are taken. These samples were then forwarded to an accredited laboratory for analysis.

**Blood Levels Found**

A blood sample taken midday from Sandra at hospital some ten hours after the offence was found to contain the 'party drug' Ecstasy 0.10 milligrams per litre, pseudoephedrine 0.05 milligrams per litre (possibly an impurity in the MDMA preparation), diazepam less than 0.1 milligrams per litre, nordiazepam less than 0.1 milligrams per litre (these indicated that a drug such as Valium had been taken sometime earlier ) – and more significantly, alcohol 0.125 grams per 100 millilitres (a decilitre) of blood.

I was asked what her blood alcohol level would have been at two a.m., about the time of the offence. I indicated that the lowest possible reading would have been 0.225 and the top end reading would have been 0.375 grams per decilitre, with a more likely reading of 0.325 grams per decilitre of blood. Whilst Sandra was a seasoned drinker of alcohol (and she apparently had a problem in this area) these were very high readings. They would account for her condition, as observed by witnesses and police, due to the alcohol alone – aside from the other drugs detected in her blood. Therefore, her ability to ward off unwanted sexual advances by Grose was, clearly, very compromised…

**The Outcome**

The magistrate found that the prosecution had failed to produce enough evidence that Ken Grose had attempted to carry out the rape, as penile penetration appeared to have not occurred. Therefore, there was insufficient evidence for a conviction over the offence – and so, he was cleared over the incident. The case was dismissed.

However, as one wag put it on leaving the Court, “He was armless but not ‘armless [harmless]!” - and he did try to ‘to get a root’. But for his disability and more so the quantity of alcohol on board, he may well have succeeded in his stated quest to the bar tender – with a very different outcome!

# 16
# The Lady in the Bath Water

*"Chains of habit are too light to be felt*
*until they are too heavy to be broken."*

Warren Buffett

## Introduction

Propofol, known to science as 2,6-diisopropylphenol, is a short-acting intravenous anaesthetic drug that is structurally unrelated to other anaesthetic agents:

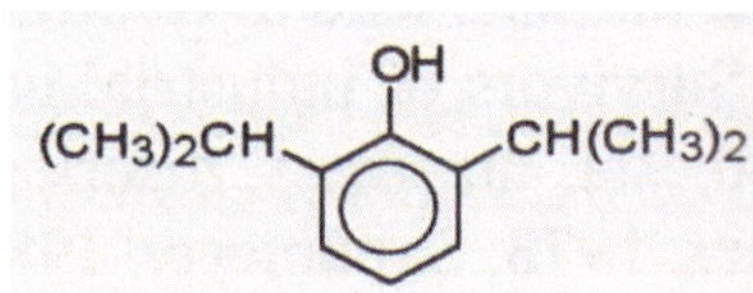


*Fig. 125: Chemical structure of propofol.*

It is available under the trade name of Diprivan and is a sedative-hypnotic which is used as a intravenous anaesthetic agent. It is available as an oil/water emulsion in 20-100 mL vials containing 10 mg/mL as the free acid.

Abuse of the anaesthetic drug propofol appears to be rare. However, it featured in the death of the American singer, Michael Jackson on June 25, 2009 – a sedative and a hospital-grade anaesthetic – which killed the superstar.

The Los Angeles County Coroner stated that, "Cause of death [of Michael Jackson] was established as acute propofol intoxication." Another sedative, lorazepam, or 'Ativan' had also contributed to his death.

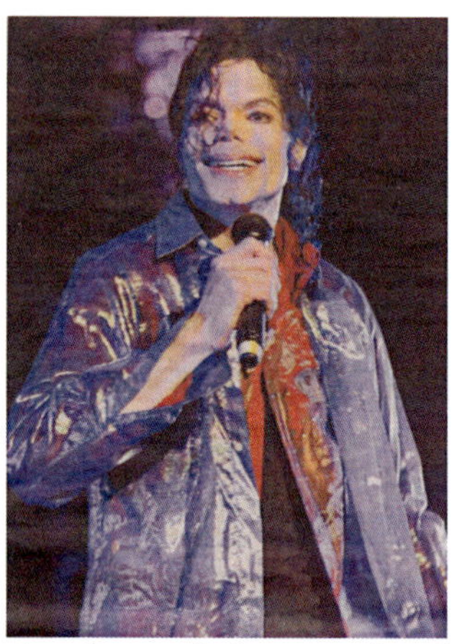

Fig. 127: *Michael Jackson in rehearsals just two days before his death. [Courtesy* Sunday Telegraph, *August 30, 2009].*

Propofol's use is characterised by a quick onset of action, a short duration of activity and a dose-dependent depth of sedation. This means essentially that the depth of anaesthesia can be induced according to the dosage given to the patient. It is well known that propofol administration, even in a therapeutic dose, can cause respiratory depression. Therefore, oxygen and respiratory assistance is generally needed, with its use being more appropriate in a hospital setting where these facilities are available.

However, euphoria, sexual hallucinations and disinhibitions have been observed with propofol anaesthesia. It is these effects which could explain the recreational use of the drug particularly with young healthcare professionals who have ready access to the drug. One female radiographer even describing the preparation as "the milk of human kindness" – before the drug, ironically, took her life.

Another similar case involved a very promising medical professional, an attractive female anaesthetics doctor in her early thirties, found dead at home in her bath after self-administration of propofol, apparently for recreational purposes. She had a number of needle marks on her body suggesting regular usage of the drug. A number of opened and unopened vials of propofol were found in her apartment, along with a cannula inserted into her arm attached to syringe – suicide, a tragic accidental death or a drug-assisted murder?

### A Troubled Love Life

Doctor Linda Goodhart (not her real name) was a well respected anaesthetist. She was very professional at her occupation and was well regarded by her colleagues and assisting nurses. Just recently, she had passed her Fellowship in Anaesthetics – and she was on her way to become a consultant. The pinnacle of her career! Linda had many friends in Sydney, although most were doctors and various other professionals. Unfortunately Linda had a troubled love life and the 'boyfriends' in her life treated her poorly, and she clearly needed a decent male relationship which would probably have been more appropriate, given her existing circle of friends. Unfortunately, one in particular, Dan (not his real name*)* who frequently attended her apartment, was into drugs and violence. On one occasion she sustained an injury to her face. "My whole eye and cheekbone is bruised seeing double," she texted to Dan. Her relationship with Dan appeared to be mainly based on sex and drugs (such as cannabis and cocaine). Unfortunately, Dan did not value her as she deserved and treated her badly. Her friends urged her to, "get out of the relationship." To further complicate things, Linda was having an affair with another doctor which caused her a "lot of emotional pain" during their time together. Amazingly, he was still seeing Linda despite being in a de facto relationship and was apparently, with Linda the weekend before he was married! One wonders how the future wife would have felt about this, had she known.

## Where is She?

Despite Dr Goodhart's troubled and complicated love life, she was a highly regarded professional who possessed great clinical skills and showed a great empathy towards her patients. So there was some surprise when she did not present herself for duty as the emergency obstetric anaesthetic registrar on the morning of 18 June, 2006. This soon turned to some concern, as the morning wore on and she failed to respond to telephone and paging calls. At ten thirty a.m. the switchboard advised Dr Howard (not his real name), another anaesthetic senior registrar, that Dr Goodhart had not arrived to work for her eight a.m. start and inquired if he knew where she was.

"This is so out of character for her not to show up for work without calling," Dr Howard recalled saying.

He then attempted to call her on her mobile and landline without success.

The consultant anaesthetist then asked Dr Howard to go to Dr Goodhart's apartment to ensure that she had not suffered any complications from her previous injury. About eleven a.m. Dr Howard arrived at Linda's apartment.

After several attempts to gain entry, he sought out the security manager for the apartments and expressed his concerns for Dr Goodhart's welfare.

## A Grim Discovery

The manager arranged for a locksmith to attend, who arrived at eleven forty-five a.m. and, eventually, entry was gained into the modest one-bedroom apartment. It contained a separate bathroom, an open area living room with a connecting kitchen and an adjoining exterior balcony. As the three men entered the apartment, they passed an area of bloodstaining on the tiled floor outside the bathroom, near an unplugged television set.

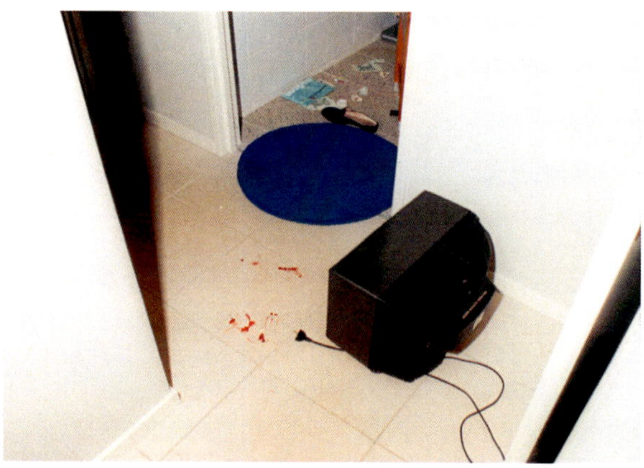

*Fig. 127: View of bloodstains on floor near television set.*

The bathroom door was ajar. On entering, a grim sight befell them: Dr Linda Goodhart's naked body was found in a foetal position partially submerged in the bathtub, and inserted in her arm was an intravenous cannula with a syringe attached, which was gently floating in the bath water…

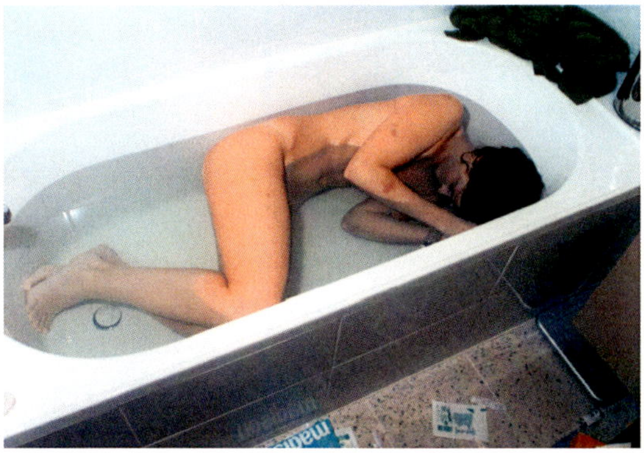

*Fig. 128: View of the deceased as she lay in the bath*

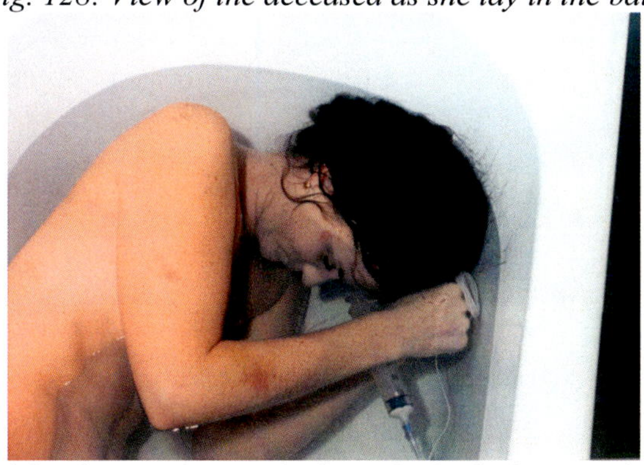

*Fig. 129: View of the deceased upper body in the bath showing the floating syringe tube*

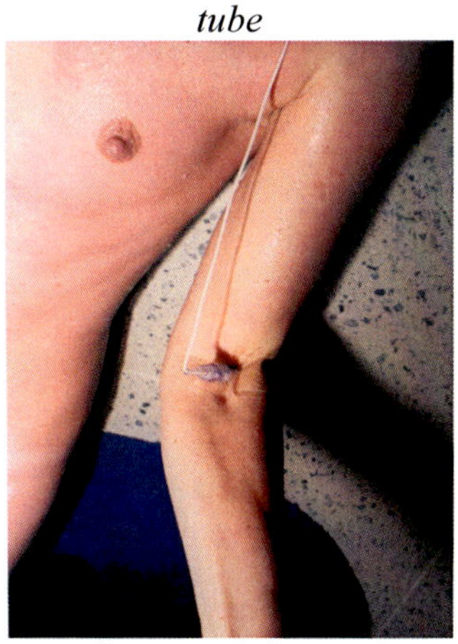

*Fig. 130: View of the deceased's inner left arm showing the cannula insertion. [Photos: Courtesy of Crime Scene, NSW Police Force.]*

Quite alarmed at this point, the locksmith reached for his mobile phone and rang for the police and an ambulance. The police arrived sometime later, and a crime scene was established. Brief statements were taken from each of the three men, and the crime scene investigation (CSI) police then examined the area and photographed various items.

On one corner of the bath were four green candle holders, containing burnt candles and there was black sooting on the tiles above these candles.

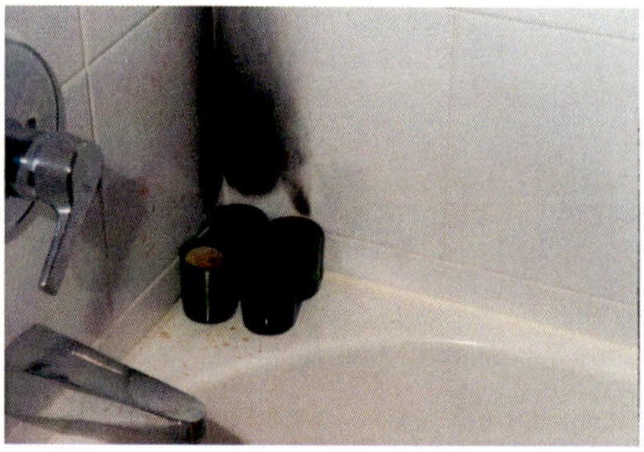

*Fig. 131: View of four green candle holders containing burnt candles.*

Nearby was a waste bin which contained a black mobile phone, an empty vial of Diprivan, wrappings and medical paraphernalia.

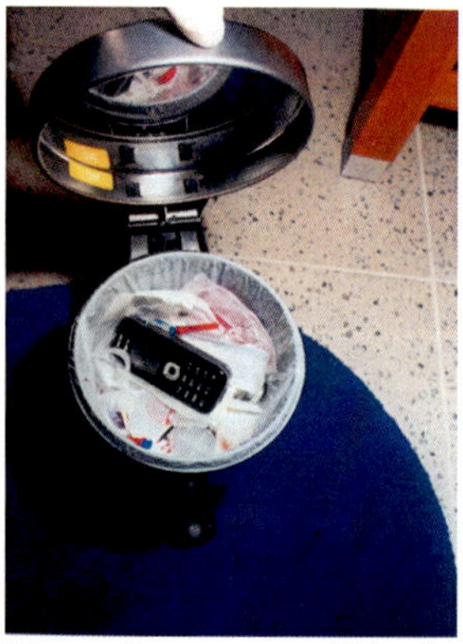

*Fig. 132: View of contents of bin found nearby*

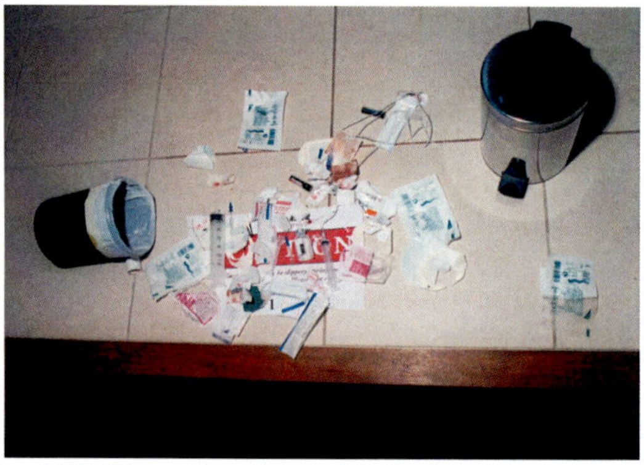

*Fig. 133: View of medical debris found in apartment*

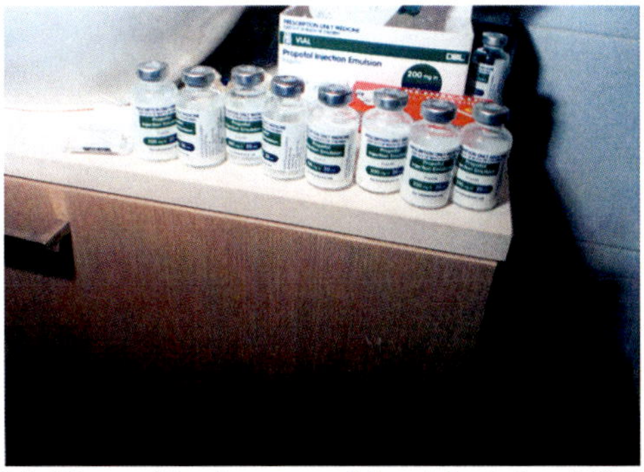

*Fig. 134: View of bathroom table with vials of 'Diprivan'*
*[Photos: Courtesy of Crime Scene, NSW Police Force]*

Further supplies of Diprivan vials were found in the bathroom and throughout the apartment:

It would appear that Dr Goodhart was ensuring she had adequate supplies of the drug, propofol, on hand. But did she commit suicide or was it an accident of recreational use that had gone terribly wrong? After her body was conveyed by Government contractors to a nearby hospital for death certification, the police team further inspected her apartment. A further two vials of propofol were found in a toiletries bag in her bedroom cupboard, along with two vibrators and numerous condoms. An accidental death appeared more likely.

Propofol may be used to induce and enhance sexual pleasure and that would suggest the latter view of recreational use.

## Blood Levels Found

A blood sample taken from the deceased doctor at the post mortem was found to have present propofol 2.6 milligrams per litre. Her urine sample was found to have present 0.8 milligrams of propofol and her bile sample 3 milligrams per litre of propofol.

For the induction of anaesthesia, blood levels of about 6-10 milligrams per litre are necessary, but during maintenance of anaesthesia levels of about 2-4 mg/L are sufficient. The level of propofol found in Dr Goodhart's blood was within this latter range, and the presence of modest levels of the drug in her urine and bile indicated she was alive for some time before she became immersed in the bath water. Therefore, assisted death or murder was unlikely.

The risk of death due to self-administered propofol intoxication is low, mainly due to the low concentration found in commercial vials (20 ml containing 200 mg propofol or 500mg/50 ml, pre-filled syringe. This is equivalent to a standard dose of 2-2.5 mg/kg body weight for the induction of general anaesthesia. The fast-acting narcotic effect of propofol (one to two minutes after injection) prevents self-injection of more than one vial at one time.

No doubt, Dr Goodhart would have been well aware of this.

However, healthcare workers such as medical and nursing staff have greater access to this drug and therefore have a greater potential to become addicted, and deaths have occurred through overdosage.

## Probable Scenario

Goodhart had used propofol regularly and enjoyed its effects – and had developed some degree of tolerance. Hence the stocks which were found in her apartment. Given her stressed environment, this may well have been her only way of achieving some degree of fulfilment both emotionally and sexually.

A probable scenario was that of a regular propofol user returning from a difficult shift and seeking some physical and mental relief. After some attempts of inserting the cannula, (hence the bloodstains in the hallway) she slipped out of her clothes and into a warm bath, lit the candles for effect, then to relax and enjoy the effects of the drug. Unfortunately, this day was going to be quite different from those previously. Possibly, being more fatigued than in previous situations, she fell asleep and her head slipped beneath the bath waters. Blissfully unaware, she would have been asleep as she drowned in her bath water.

The pathologist wrote in his report, "The presence of pulmonary oedema and generalised organ congestion is consistent with both administration of an overdose of a respiratory depressant agent and death due to immersion."

I wrote in my statement that, "It would appear that the propofol was self-administered, probably recreationally, resulting in respiratory depression and consequent anoxia with the possibility of immersion, resulting in her death." I had to agree with the pathologist that death was due to immersion essentially, drowning. However, the "level of propofol present in her blood in an apparently tolerant person, does not appear to be excessive, though quite sufficient to result in central nervous system depression."

Therefore, whilst asleep this deadly combination of anaesthesia due to propofol, drowning was to take her life.

## Conclusion

It is an unfortunate trait of humans to resort to substance abuse to relieve stress from overwork and/or poor relationships: sexual or otherwise. A subsequent inquest found that this was an accidental death. In this case the drug, propofol, contributed to snuffing out the life of a promising young medical professional, like the flames of the candles found in her bathroom.

As Sir Elton John so eloquently put it, in his song about the death of a young movie legend of comparable age, Marilyn Monroe:

"She lived her life like a candle in the wind…"

And so, it appeared, did the good doctor.

# 17
# The 'Cheese Ball' Killer – The Car as a Murder Weapon

*"Before you embark on a journey of revenge, dig two graves."*

Confucius, China's most famous teacher,
philosopher and political theorist (551-479 BC)

### A Night out with Friends

Eli Westlake, was a very likeable young man of twenty-one years and was said to be a promising young musician, a 'bit of character' and he was the son of composer, Nigel Westlake. Eli was very close to his elder brother, Joel Westlake.

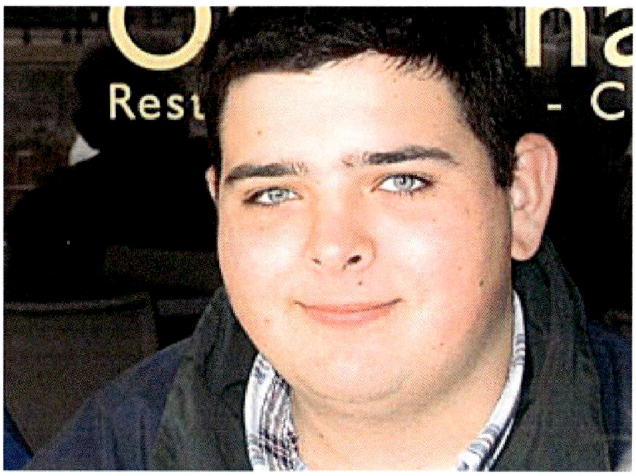


Fig. 135. Eli Westlake.
*[Source:* The Daily Telegraph, *March 26, 2010*]

On 6 June 2008 he went to his brother's home and joined him and a group of friends recording music and drinking. Apparently this was a regular event as Eli was establishing himself as a DJ on the Kings Cross nightclub scene. They left Joel's home after two thirty a.m. and went to the St Leonard's Tavern to continue drinking and enjoying one another's company. In the early hours of June 7, 2008 Eli Westlake was walking home from St Leonards Tavern with his older brother, Joel Westlake and some friends, Jesse Horn and Toby Finlayson. Just after four .a.m. they went into a 7-Eleven convenience store and Joel Westlake bought a pack of cheese and bacon balls. This purchase was to play a much larger part in the subsequent events than it should have been in normal circumstances.

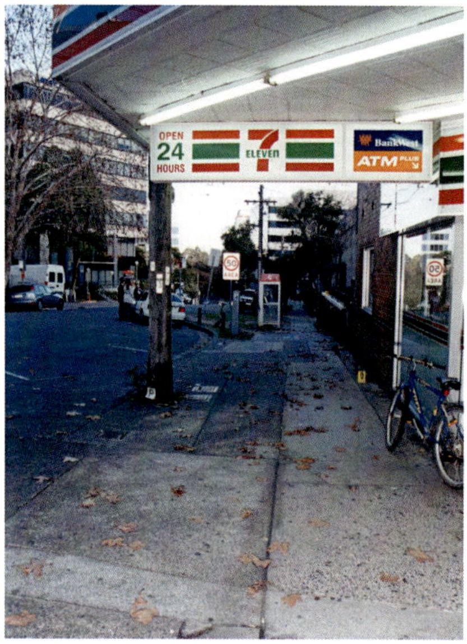


*Fig. 136. The 7-Eleven store where the cheese balls were purchased.*

Meanwhile, Sarah May Ward was also enjoying an evening with her companion, William Long and friends, Anthony Gilbert and Lisa Polombi at Mr Gilbert's home in Artarmon. She smoked two cones of cannabis, consumed a bottle of wine and had taken four five-milligram tablets of Valium (her regular dose was two tablets per day). She then travelled with the group to the Sebel Apartments and then at about eleven p.m., onto the Monkey Bar at Chatswood. At that time she took an Ecstasy tablet which was washed down with a glass of wine. She and her friends then returned to Artarmon at about midnight. Anthony Gilbert and Lisa Polombi watched television for a time with Sarah Ward and William Long before going to bed. Sarah and William, known as Bill, stayed up watching television and she drank another bottle of wine…

At about four a.m. the pair made the fateful decision to drive Anthony Gilbert's Toyota Lexcen (UOX-230) to St Leonards. At about four twenty a.m., they arrived at Christie Lane, St Leonards where they encountered Eli Westlake, his older brother, Joel Westlake and their friends, Jesse Horn and Toby Finlayson. Eli was in a playful mood, and on seeing the couple in the vehicle, reached into the bag of cheese balls and threw some of them into the air like confetti "as a celebratory gesture", and shouted, "Happy honeymoon!"

Some of the cheese balls landed on the car's bonnet and into the vehicle. Ms Ward was not impressed. She got out of the vehicle in a "very aggressive" mood and tried to hit Eli's brother, Joel, then tried to punch and kick Toby Finlayson who cried out, "Settle down, it's just chips. What are you doing?" in an effort to defuse the situation.

The group thought that was the end of the incident, as they moved down the alleyway and away from the vehicle.

Unfortunately, a dreadful tragedy was about to unfold.

## Enter the Predator

In the meantime, Ms Ward had got back into the car and sat in the driver's seat fuming, while Mr Long sat in the passenger seat, and after a while she said, "I have had enough of these guys".

She then hit the accelerator and drove the vehicle in an erratic manner to Lithgow Street, where Eli Westlake and others of the group were walking.

Unfortunately, Eli Westlake was quite distinguishable from the group by the white 'Sloppy Joe' he was wearing which stood out in the car headlights. Ward drove toward the group, hitting Eli on the legs as he tried to get out of the way.

"What did you do that for?" he cried out, limping away from the scene.

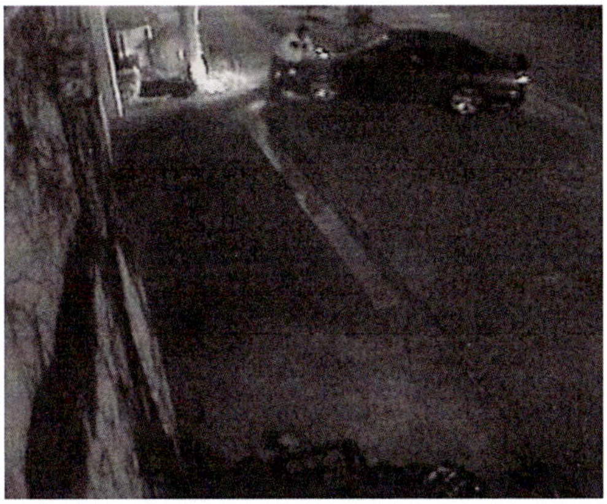

*Fig. 137. Ms Ward's first attempt on Eli Westlake's life, captured on a CC TV camera outside the Cabana Bar, North Sydney.*

Toby Finlayson realising things were getting out of hand, shouted out to his friends, "Run, let's get out of here. This is crazy."

The friends then took off and hid in fear behind the industrial skip bins in the street.

Ward reversed the vehicle and then turned off the lights, lying in waiting.

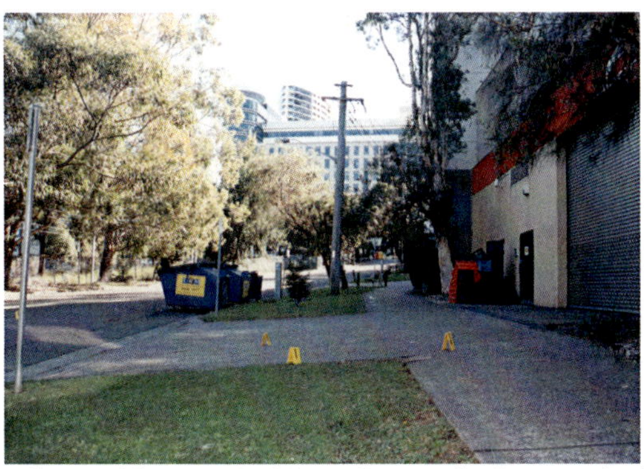

*Fig. 138.The industrial bins in Lithgow Street, St. Leonards that provided a temporary 'safe haven' at the time of the incident.*

After a short time, thinking the danger was over, Eli Westlake and Jesse Horne emerged from their cover only to be greeted by a high beam flash of headlights. The car lunged forward. It was too late to run.

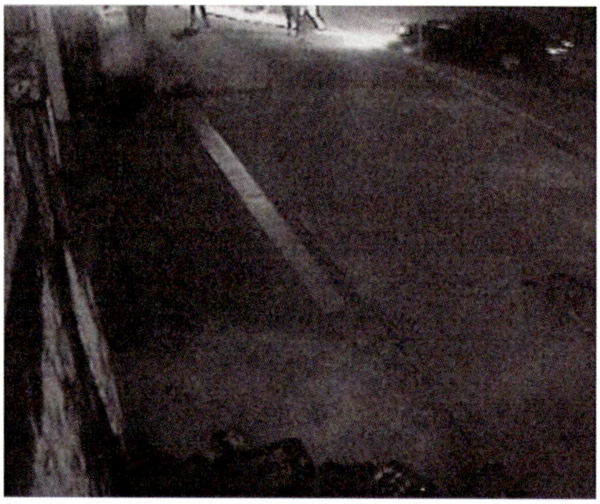

*Fig. 139. Ms Ward's second attempt on Eli Westlake's life, captured on a CC TV camera outside the Cabana Bar, North Sydney. This time, she hit him again with the motor vehicle resulting in fatal injuries.*

Just like an unfortunate rabbit caught in the headlights of an oncoming motor vehicle, the car drove over the kerb, crossing a grassed nature strip and hit the leg of Jesse Horne, who went up over the bonnet and landed on the kerb. Fortunately he suffered only minor injuries as a result of the impact.

Toby Finlayson checked his friend and found he was okay, aside from bruising to the right side of his body and lacerations on his hands from the windscreen wipers.

Eli Westlake was not so lucky. He had been knocked down by the impact and his body pinned under the car, as the vehicle careered down a set of stairs at the entrance of 67 Lithgow Street to the Oxygen gym and on to a tiled floor at the bottom of the stairs. The vehicle came to rest on the stairwell on top of Eli's body, resulting in fatal injuries.

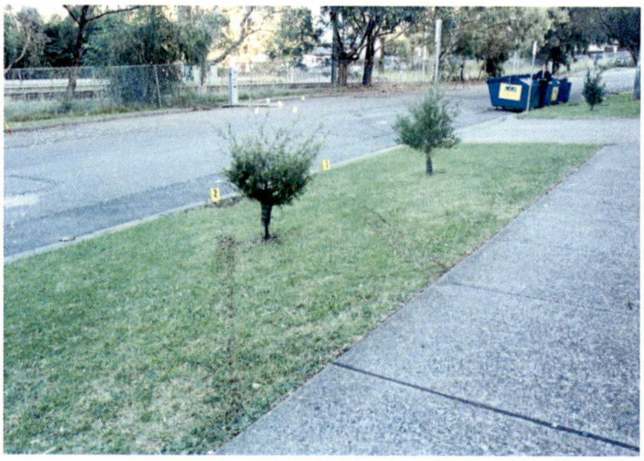

*Fig. 140. The grassy nature strip where the vehicle driven by Sarah Ward impacted upon Jesse Horne and Eli Westlake.*

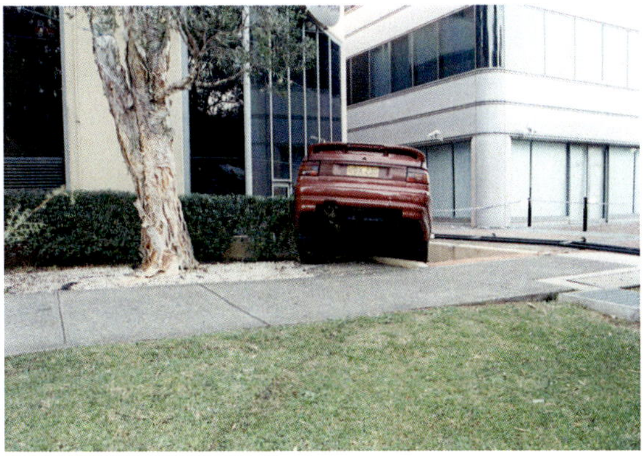

*Fig. 141...and the maroon Toyota Lexcen murder 'weapon' vehicle.*

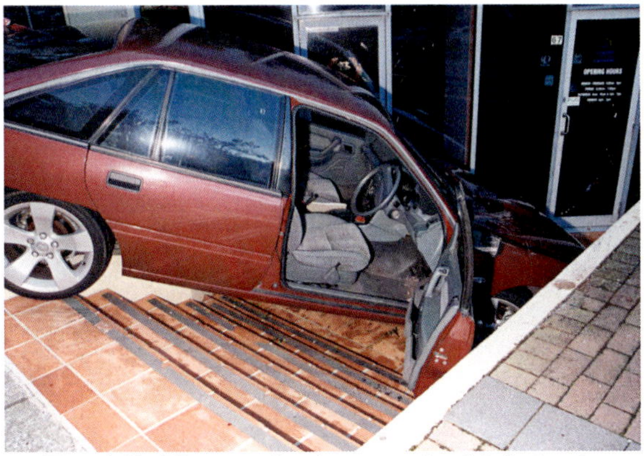

*Fig. 142. The murder 'weapon' vehicle in situ*

Mr Long exited the vehicle and fled from the scene, while Sarah Ward got out of the vehicle and stayed at the scene. Police and an ambulance were called.

At the time, no one realised Eli was under the assault vehicle where he was either dying or already dead.

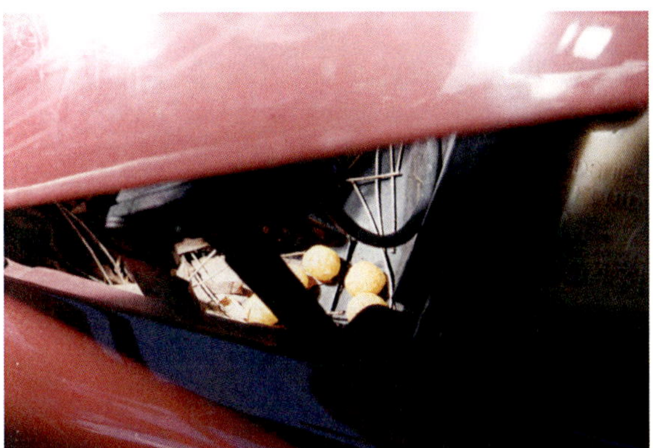

*Fig. 143. Some of the 'offending' cheese balls remaining in the vehicle.*

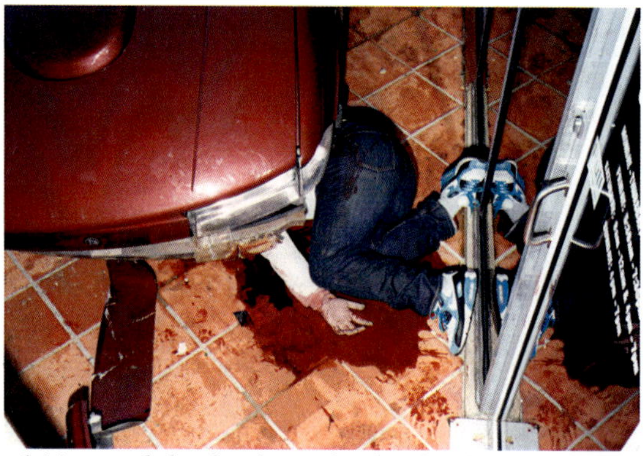

*Fig. 144....and the fatal result, the death of Eli Westlake.*
*[Photographs: Sydney Crime Scene, NSW Police Force.]*

The predatory assault was successful. But the fallout from the incident proved to be devastating: a promising young life snuffed out and a not-so-young life, possibly damaged beyond repair...

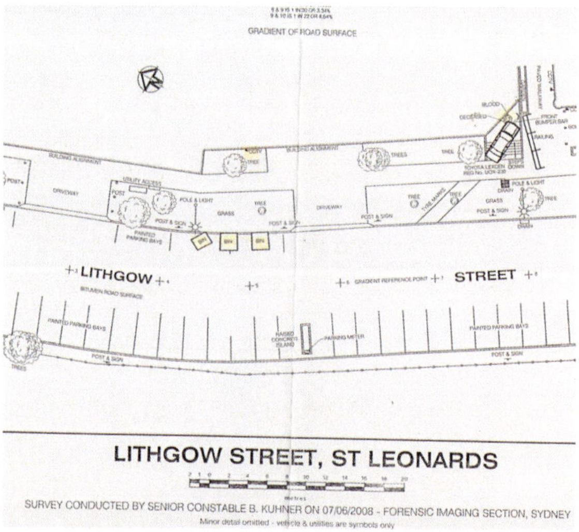


*Fig. 145. A crime scene diagram of Lithgow Street, St Leonards, where the fatal event took place.*
*[Source: Forensic Imaging Section, NSW Police Force.]*

## The Darkest Hour is Just Before Dawn

Eli's brother was one of the first on the scene, and held the hand of his dying brother trying to comfort him, "Please help. My brother's been killed."

His friends then gathered together to lift the vehicle off the now deceased, without success. The police and ambulance officers arrived a short time later.

Joel Westlake, now aware that his brother was dead, in anger mixed with grief, turned to one of the police officers and said, "That's my fucking brother he is dead – and that bitch killed him" He was pointing at Sarah Ward, who now appeared in a hysterical state.

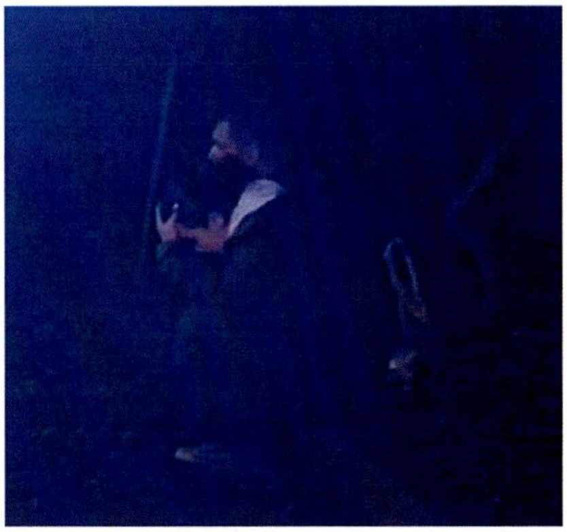

*Fig. 146. Early morning grief: Eli Westlake's friends mourning his death.*

Sarah was subjected to a breath test on an Alcolizer 11653 which recorded a positive reading of 0.196, and she was arrested.

She then asked the arresting police officer, Constable Glenn Hockley, several times "Is he dead?" adding, "I think I killed him."

To which he replied, "I don't know, just take a seat in the back."

Various formalities were then carried out, before Sarah Ward was conveyed to Chatswood Police Station for the purpose of a breath analysis. She underwent a breath analysis and 'returned a positive reading of 0.145 grammes of alcohol per 100 millilitres of blood.' Given the circumstances, it was now necessary to also get a blood and urine sample from Ms Ward. She was then taken to Royal North Shore Hospital for this procedure to be carried out. Her blood sample was taken by Dr Earl Abraham and urine sample by Nurse Wanda O'Grady at six thirty a.m. This time was important in determining her degree of intoxication at the time of the event, which fortunately was recorded by the CC TV camera at about four twenty-eight a.m. An accurate back calculation was now possible.

Dawn had now long passed, and the carnage was now evident, when vehicle UOX-230 was removed by crane at one fifty-five p.m. revealing Eli Westlake's body in its entirety. He was lying on his right side with his legs bent up in front of his torso and his left arm stretched out front of his body. There was an extensive amount of blood over his head, and this blood had pooled around his body. This blood appeared to come from his nose, mouth and right ear, indicating extensive cranial injuries.

About two oh five p.m. Eli Westlake's body was conveyed to Royal North Shore Hospital where a life extinct certificate was issued by Dr Jeremy Pallot. His body was then conveyed to Glebe Morgue for examination, and to establish the extent of his injuries sustained in the incident which had resulted in his death.

In the meantime, Sarah Ward was in Police custody and taken away for questioning.

It had been an evening which had gone very "pear shaped" for all parties concerned.

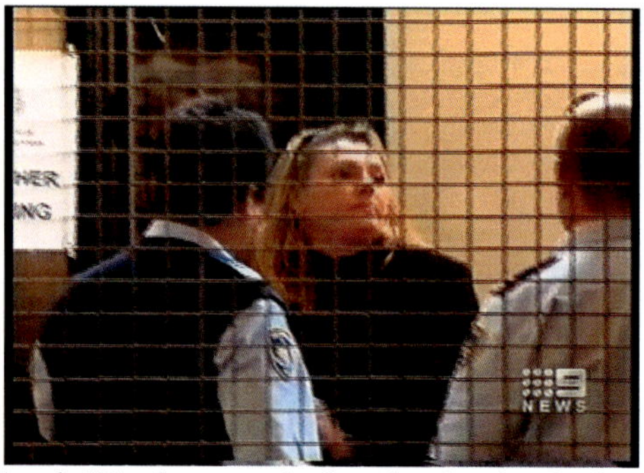


Fig. 147. Sarah Ward arrested after the death of Elias Westlake.
[*Source:* Channel 9 News]

**The ERISP Interview**

Today, the majority of Police interviews are electronically recorded, including audio and video. This evidence can then be replayed using the in-court displays and sound reinforcement systems. At the time of writing, over 160 courtrooms are now ERISP (Electronic Recorded Interviews of Suspected People) compliant. Defence lawyers are not very happy about this as they cannot raise doubt that the Police have in some way behaved inappropriately during the interview. Interviews, including the one carried out with Sarah Ward, which have been video-recorded also have the added benefit of permitting the Court to see for themselves the facial expressions and body language of the accused person. This case was no exception, the CCTV footage along with the ERISP proved to be very valuable for the prosecution.

Sarah Ward was taken to Chatswood Police Station for interview on the 7 June, 2008 by Detective Senior Constable Matthew Harmer. After the usual protocols, explanation of rights and various other details including names of participants and age of the interviewee, the interview commenced to determine what had happened and possible reasons for the incident to unfold.

The following are excerpts from that interview:

**Q.** 'Sarah, just what I'll like you to do first of all, is just go back to yesterday OK and just tell me what happened yesterday, starting in the morning going through until you're arriving here and where we are now.'

***A.*** 'OK I was at my friend's Anthony's, I was having wine, drinking, and we, a friend, myself went to St Leonards to the supermarket there to get a packet of cigarettes. When we turned up there, as soon as we turned up, there were these guys and they, and, and just attacked us, and I wasn't driving then. Then we, and then we went… we got out to get some cigarettes, and these guys, I dunno where they came from, they just sort of, and they had words and words that were said back at them, I dunno how many there, and they just sort of jumped my, us and myself and another gentleman, the gentleman I was with, and we tried to get back into the car and I got to the driver's seat, the driver's seat and he, the driver's, we got, we got it, he got to the passenger's, and I was, dunno, going, trying to get out there really, and, but driving, trying to get out of the lane in the street still, and I think it goes to, with the railway there, and I was driving the gentleman who I was with, there was, these other people were around and I'm trying to drive and get out of it and he grabbed the wheel and I went veering up into the side to somewhere and that's when I hit someone. Then I jumped out there was someone underneath the car, I tried to reverse, I couldn't get out, I tried to get the car up, I tried, I couldn't get him out, now he's dead. I was never meant to… tell it how it happened or why at how it happened.'

So much for how the events unfolded. It would have been impossible to reverse the car as the rear wheels were no longer in contact with the ground!

The interview then moved onto determining how much alcohol was consumed and when it was consumed. This information was important to determine her degree of impairment and/or intoxication at the time of the incident:

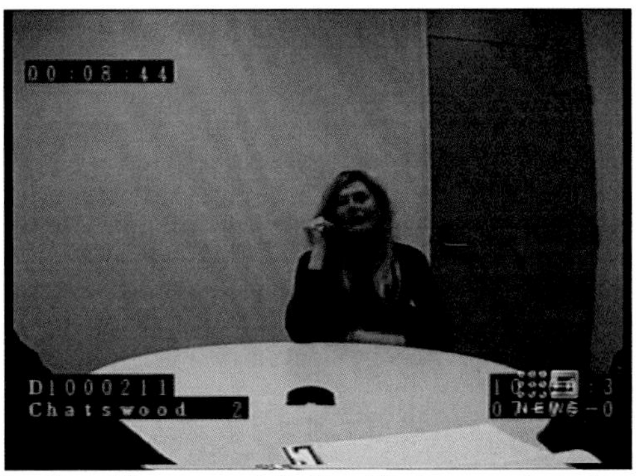


*Fig. 148. Sarah Ward at Chatswood Police Station undergoing an Electronically Recorded Interview with Detective Senior Constable Matthew Harmer. Source: Police ERISP footage and Channel 9 News*

**Q.** 'How much wine did you drink?'

**A.** 'About… I had a bottle of wine that I shared with Lisa before we left and went to the Monkey Bar.'

**Q.** 'That was before you went out?'

**A.** 'And then I had a glass of, and wine at the Monkey Bar, and then I bought a bottle of wine to, to take away from there and then I went back, [SNIFFING] pardon me, I drank that.'

**Q.** 'You drank that at Anthony's when you got home? Drinking it to yourself or did you share it with the others?'
**A.** 'Lisa might have had half a glass of it'

**Q.** 'And did you finish that bottle or..? Yes?'
**A.** 'Yes.'

**Q.** 'OK and so you're at home drinking, you… was Anthony up drinking with you?'
**A.** 'For a while, then he fell asleep.'

**Q.** 'Yes, and you said previously that Lisa had gone to sleep as well?'
**A.** 'Yeah, Lisa…'

**Q.** 'So what were you and this unknown male doing after the other two?'
**A.** 'Sitting, talking.'

**Q.** 'Yes, and how long?'
**A.** 'About an hour or so I think.'

**Q.** 'Yeah, yes?'

Then the fateful decision was made to go out after a session of drinking…

***A.*** 'And, and then we wanted to get cigarettes… Ran out of cigarettes, I never would've, I wish I never walked out the door.'

**Q.** 'So you wanted cigarettes, you went out. Did you go by yourself or with this other bloke?'
**A.** 'I went with the other to, with the gentleman.' [later identified as Bill Long]

**Q.** 'Yeah. So you went out and how did you get to the cigarettes?'

Sarah Ward then describes how they borrowed keys to their friend's car to go out and buy cigarettes from a 7-Eleven store in St Leonards, prior to their encounter with Eli Westlake and his friends…

***A.*** 'And into that street and, and, and we just pulled and we sort of pulled in and all of a sudden there were like five guys came out and they were abusing this guy, having a go at him, and hitting the window and I got out, we both got out actually, and they were sort of… they were just sort of… they were abusing us and then…'

**Q.** 'How…?'
**A.** '… pushed us and…'

**Q.** 'How do you mean, what were they doing? You said they were banging on the window and having a go?'

**A.** 'Yeah, at the driver's window, they were hitting the driver's window and carrying on and then I got out and the he's got pulverised, and then we jumped into the car. But I got into the driver's just to get out of there, then I went down the street and they were all, there were heaps of them down the street. I'm trying to turn but I shouldn't have, but I turned around and then…'

**Q.** 'OK just stop. Did you go into the shop?'

**A.** 'No, we didn't get to the shop.'

Further questions were raised concerning the incident, and Ms Ward provided various explanations for her behaviour and the alleged aggressive actions of the young men directed at her and her partner, and efforts that were taken to leave the scene…

**Q.** 'All right, so you go down this street and…'

**A.** 'Then I was going like I was going fast, I just wanted to get out of there and turn, I was trying to going and doing a U-ey or something, turn around and go up 'cause I saw them all down, they were all, there were heaps of them on the street, and then the guy I was with, he grabbed the wheel and I just fuckin' veering off and he hit this guy on the road and it killed him… I couldn't even believe it, I didn't know anyone was there when I got out and reversing back, and the big… there was a, the big guy that hit me a few times, he goes, my mate's under the car. And I got out and I…'

**Q.** 'The street where you hit him is the next street over, can you tell me how you got into Lithgow Street from where you were?

**A.** 'The street where I hit him?'

Ms Ward seemed unable to provide a satisfactory explanation to how the vehicle ended up in the street where the incident took place, and the possibility that a 'male grabbed the wheel' causing the vehicle to veer off the road.

**Q.** 'When the male grabbed the wheel and you started veering, did you stop the car? Did you try and stop the car, what'd you do?'

**A.** 'Yeah, I went down into an embankment and…'

**Q.** 'OK. But when he grabbed the wheel, did you make any attempt to stop the car?'

**A.** 'Yeah, I tried to stop it.'

**Q.** 'What did you do?'

**A.** 'I think I put the brakes on, I can't remember, I can't remember, I mean you're telling me I was in another street now…'

Further questions were asked in relation to the incident, and then moved on to formalising the identification of the driver and passenger involved in the 'indictable offence.' After some questioning, it was established that Ms Ward was the driver at the time of the offence, and that she had never seen the young men involved in a previous 'alleged altercation'. By this time, Sarah Ward was getting somewhat emotional, possibly on realising the enormity of the situation.

Detective Senior Constable Harmer left briefly to get some tissues for Sarah, while Detective Senior Constable Lawson continued the necessary formalities.

**Q.** 'It's the seventh of the sixth 2008 and it's…'
**A.** 'It could have been my son… I tried, I tried to… I tried to push the car up but, I tried so hard to stay out of trouble.'

The interview was suspended at this point due to time constraints. A further interview was carried out at one fifty-four p.m., Saturday, 7 June, 2008 with Detective Senior Constables, Matthew Harmer and Scott Lawson. This time, the footage from the CCTV was shown to Ms Ward…

**Q.** 'The time by this CCTV down the bottom here, it says four twenty-five, 04.25.02 and the date being 2008, 06 being the month of June and 07 being the seventh, today's date. This footage is starting just when you first come in contact in Lithgow Street.'
**A.** 'Where have I gone?'

**Q.** 'You can see the headlights here, the car's just over this, just off the screen there. So you agree the car drove up just a minute ago and struck a male by the legs, the car reversed backwards.'
**A.** 'Yeah, is that the man I killed?'

**Q.** 'No.'
**A.** 'I, I hit two people.'

Detective Senior Constable Harmer then took her through the CCTV footage with the assistance of Detective Senior Constable Lawson…

**Q.** 'Just at that time when you just saw that video, Sarah, was the guy Bill, was he in the car at that time as well?'
**A.** 'Yes, he was in the car.'

**Q.** 'And do you believe that where you saw the car there, can you explain, you said before that the steering wheel was grabbed by Bill?'
**A.** 'To, yeah, to get, to try and turn me around but I wasn't, I couldn't drive. I couldn't get it into reverse I had these boots on and I couldn't turn around and I hit the accelerator and I couldn't stop and I went through down an embankment or something, I didn't even know someone was under there till someone screaming

and said, someone was there and I just got out and I tried to lift the car up and I…'

Further questions were raised to establish her drinking history and any drugs and/or medications she was taking. It was established that she consumed a number of drugs including an Ecstasy' tablet:

**A.** 'I had one Ecstasy tablet.'

**Q.** 'When did you have that?'
**A.** 'That evening.'

**Q.** 'Along with various other drugs such as cannabis?
**A.** 'I smoke pot.'

**Q.** 'Did you smoke any yesterday?'… 'How much of it?'
**A.** 'I had about three cones in the afternoon evening early evening.'

**Q.** 'And alcohol?'
**A.** 'I have a problem with alcohol.'

**Q.** 'You have a problem with alcohol?'
**A.** 'I binge drink… I, I drink two bottles on my own, I can drink two… wine…'

Detective Senior Constable Harmer then took this line of questioning further.

**Q.** 'And how do you, say, after drinking a couple of bottles of wine, you would be intoxicated… well intoxicated or moderate or…?'
**A.** 'I don't know. Sometimes I can handle it, sometimes I can't.'

**Q.** 'What happens to you when you can't?'
**A.** 'I suppose I can get emotional and fight. I've done it all", (but not recently)'

- along with various other drugs such as anti-depressants, 'coke' (cocaine),before the interview was concluded.

**Eli Westlake's Post Mortem**

The post mortem of Eli Westlake was carried out by Dr Rianie Janse Van Vuuren at 0900 hours on 8 June 2008. He was only twenty-one years old.

Part of the post mortem report described the following:

"External post-mortem examination showed multiple bruises and abrasions to the body, both on the anterior and posterior surfaces. There was an almost linear abrasion to the head and the left posterior aspect of the head appeared deformed.

There were petechial haemorrhages in the eyes and on the right arm, probably position dependent. The right hand had a washerwomen's appearance, which could be related to the post-mortem position. The mandible had a fracture of the right lateral aspect."

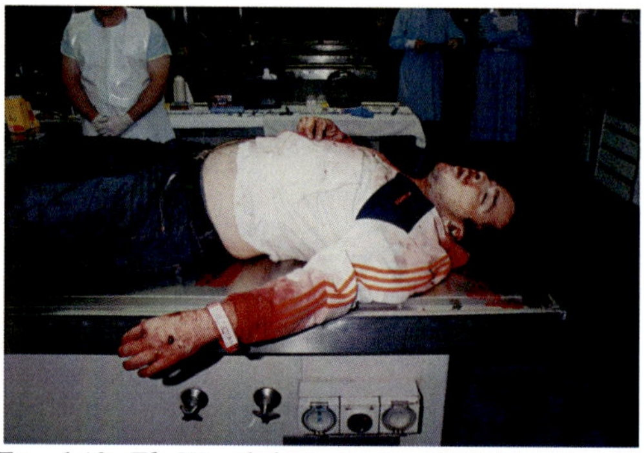

*Fig. 149. Eli Westlake's body at Glebe morgue.*
*[Source: Sydney Crime Scene, NSW Police Force]*

Eli's body had clearly been knocked about when the car impacted with him the second time. But more importantly, were the severe head injuries he sustained in the onslaught.

These head injuries were itemised as follows:

- *Base of skull fractures extending into temporal bones on both sides,*
- *Subarachnoid haemorrhages on brain,*
- *Cerebral swelling with parahippocampal gyrus herniation,*
- *Laceration to left uncus,*
- *Left optic nerve laceration,*
- *Multiple haemorrhages in floor of fourth ventricle and in pons.*

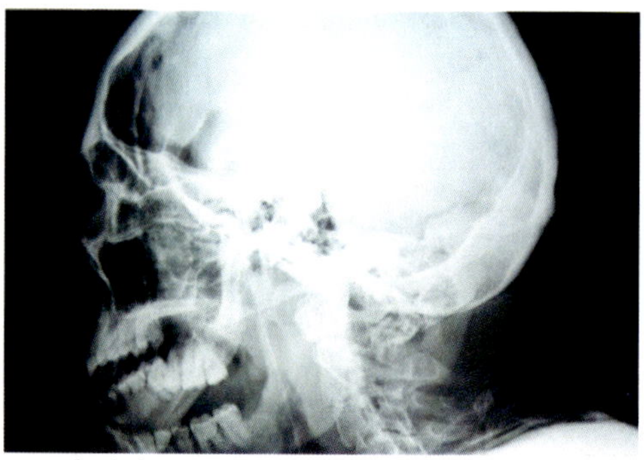

*Fig. 150. An X-ray revealed the extent of the injuries sustained by Eli Westlake when the vehicle driven by Sarah Ward impacted upon his body. Death was through extensive skull fractures and loss of blood.*

Also, his toxicological examination, "showed a high level of alcohol in the blood, with a higher level in the vitreous and highest in the urine. This would suggest that the alcohol metabolism was in the excretory phase."
These alcohol results were as follows:
Blood * Urine Vitreous humour
(preserved) (preserved)

Alcohol
0.186 g/100 ml 0.242 g/100 ml 0.219 g/100 ml

[* No other drugs were detected]

With a high range PCA (prescribed content alcohol) in his blood, Eli Westlake was well and truly intoxicated. This level of intoxication may have accounted for his playful, if not boisterous, behaviour on the night where he threw the cheese balls onto the vehicle driven by Sarah Ward, and subsequent events which led to his death.

**On Trial for Murder**

At a committal hearing for Ms Sarah Ward at Sydney's Central Local Court beginning on July 6, 2009, she appeared before Magistrate David Armati accused of murder, or on alternative counts, aggravated dangerous driving occasioning death or dangerous driving occasioning death.

Ms Sally Traynor, for the Director of Public Prosecutions outlined the events of the night of June 6, 2008, and described how Eli Westlake, his brother Joel and a group of friends were recording music and drinking at his brother's home.

At about two thirty a.m. they left and went to the St Leonard's Tavern to continue drinking. At just after four a.m., some of them went into a 7-Eleven convenience store where Joel Westlake purchased a pack of cheese balls. While walking down Christie Lane (off Lithgow Street, St Leonards) the group encountered a Toyota Lexcen sedan, driven by Ms Ward with a male companion, William 'Bill' Long. For a lark, Eli Westlake threw some of the cheese balls at the vehicle allegedly saying, "Happy honeymoon."

When the tragic events occurred as described earlier.

A number of witnesses came forward and gave evidence in relation to this matter, including myself. I was amongst the last to give evidence, and was there to interpret the levels of drugs and alcohol detected in Ms Ward's blood samples and so determine how much she would have been affected at the time of the incident. The analyst's reports, carried out by the Division of Analytical Laboratories, Lidcombe, New South Wales, showed that she had the following levels of drugs and alcohol in her blood on 7 June, 2008 at six thirty a.m.:

- 3,4-methylenedioxymethylamphetamine ('Ecstasy') 0.07 milligrams per litre,
- delta-9-tetrahydrocannabinol (delta-9-THC) 0.005 milligrams per litre,
- delta-9-THC acid 0.023 milligrams per litre,
- diazepam 0.22 milligrams per litre,

- nordiazepam 0.07 milligrams per litre,
- temazepam <0.01 milligrams per litre, and
- venlafaxine <0.1 milligrams per litre.

But more importantly was the level of alcohol present in her blood:

- alcohol 0.140 grams per decilitre (100 millilitres) of blood.

Whilst the level of cannabis detected was significant, along with the presence of diazepam, the 'major player' was alcohol. I estimated that the level of alcohol in her blood at the time of the incident most likely at 0.171% and concluded that Ms Ward "was under the combined influence of alcohol and cannabis, with probable additive effects from diazepam, to the extent that her driving ability would have been substantially impaired."

A similar estimation of her blood alcohol at the time of the incident was confirmed by another expert involved in this matter, Dr Graham Starmer, Sydney University, who considered, "that Ms Ward's most likely blood alcohol concentration at the time of the collision would have been 0.176 g/100 ml (range 0.166-0.197 g/100 ml). This is in reasonable accord with Dr Allender's estimate."

However, the most damning evidence was from the CCTV footage. There was now more than sufficient evidence for the matter to go to trial.

On 23 November, 2009 Sarah May Ward stood trial in the NSW Supreme Court at Taylor Square, Darlinghurst before Justice Roderick Howie for the murder Eli Westlake on the morning of the 7 July, 2008.

Ms Sarah Ward pleaded not guilty to murdering Mr Eli Westlake, in the early hours of June 7, 2008, in the northern Sydney suburb of St. Leonards.

The Crown would not accept Ms Ward's guilty plea to the lesser charge of manslaughter.

Prosecutor Elizabeth Wilkins SC said Sarah Ward had used "her car as a weapon" when she drove onto the footpath in pursuit of Eli Westlake.

CCTV footage of the incident showed, "this was a deliberate, controlled and predatory act by Ms Ward", said Ms Wilkins.

Ms Ward's barrister, Mr Eugene Wasilenia, said his client never intended killing or seriously injuring Mr Eli Westlake, noting that her blood alcohol reading had been 0.171 at the time of the incident, more than three times the legal limit, and that she also had drugs in her system. He contended that Ms Ward was earlier attacked by some of Eli Westlake's friends, she was unfamiliar with the borrowed car, and had been trying to get away from the scene. He said that Ms Ward had trouble reversing the car and had hit the accelerator in panic, as her passenger (Mr Long) pulled the steering wheel to get the car under control, before it hit Mr Westlake.

However, Ms Wilkins said Ms Ward *twice* aimed the car at the pedestrian in the white 'Sloppy Joe', reversing and trying again after Eli Westlake jumped out of the way after the first attempt.

She continued, "The Crown case is that the accused, on both occasions, drove her motor car up onto the footpath in order to hit him."

Ms Wilkins further stated, that as the group walked off, Ms Ward "was actually following, stalking these boys in her car, driving down a one-way street the wrong way.

"The Crown says this is one case where actions speak so much louder than words."

Then turning to the jury, Ms Wilkins said, "When you watch the CCTV, you would be satisfied this was a deliberate, controlled and predatory act by the accused… She was using her car as a weapon.

"She was out seeking revenge for what she perceived was the humiliation she suffered in the laneway."

A number of other issues were also raised during the trial, including Ms Ward's drug usage, depression, bipolar disorder and possible psychological condition.

But a Crown witness, forensic psychiatrist Dr Allnutt, said she should still have been able to "control herself," as she showed no evidence of mania at the time of the incident.

"In your view, you do not believe that – absent alcohol, which the jury must disregard – her capacity to understand or judge her actions from right or wrong, or to control, was substantially impaired?" asked Justice Howie.

"True," Dr Allnut replied.

The defence barrister, Mr Eugene Wasilenia put to the court that the incident should be considered "a chance encounter, an instantaneous reaction to a series of events, and not a premeditated attack on Mr Westlake."

He continued, "That of all the young men present that night Mr Westlake was not the most deserving or worthy of her anger."

This last comment, and the stress of the proceedings, proved to be too much for Eli's father, Nigel Westlake. He stood up and stormed out of the courtroom. Only to be followed a short time later by his other son, Joel, who swore at Mr Wasilenia, as he departed with his father.

Justice Howie told the family of Mr Westlake to talk to the pair and remind them Ms Ward was entitled to a defence, as he adjourned the hearing.

**The Verdict and Sentence**

After a trial lasting almost four weeks the NSW Supreme Court jury, by a majority verdict, found that Ms Sarah May Ward was guilty of murdering Eli Westlake. Ms Ward sat in the dock sobbing as the jury delivered this verdict after a second day of deliberations.

Justice Howie commented that Ms Ward had been the aggressor by using her car as a weapon and that none of the young men had been in any way responsible for Eli Westlake's death.

"I have no doubt that she waited on the street until the deceased ventured out of hiding.

"She was aware that, when affected by alcohol, she acted impulsively, toward things that irritated her… and that it was a senseless act of anger."

He continued that it had been Ms Ward's intention to cause serious harm to Eli Westlake, but she had not intended to kill him.

"She clearly wanted to teach the young man a lesson. It was an intention to inflict very serious injury and the risk of death was very high."

Justice Howie adding, "I accept that almost immediately she regretted her actions."

Ms Ward had apparently shown remorse by trying to help Eli Westlake's friends lift the car off him.

Justice Howie then sentenced Ms Ward to a maximum of twenty five years gaol. With time in custody, she would be eligible for parole in March, 2027.

**Aftermath**

However, the sentence handed down proved to be no comfort for the Westlake family. Outside court, Eli Westlake's father, Nigel Westlake, said his family "had been sentenced to a lifetime of anguish.

"She set upon our boys and their friends and she didn't let up until she'd killed Eli.

"No courtroom can bring back Eli, no sentence can relieve the pain of our loss. The notion of justice has very little meaning for us because the worst has already happened. Eli is taken and nothing will bring him back. We struggle each day to come to terms with this fact.

"We've heard all the evidence, seen the CCTV footage of the night in question and we concur with the findings of the jury, as tragic as this is not only for us but for the family of the accused and the accused herself."

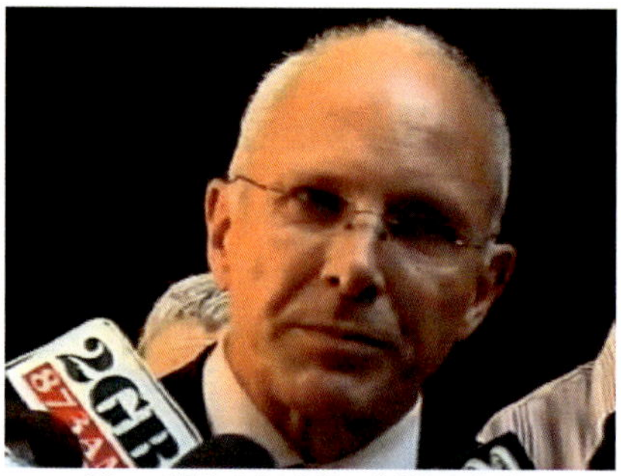

*Fig. 151 Mr. Nigel Westlake*

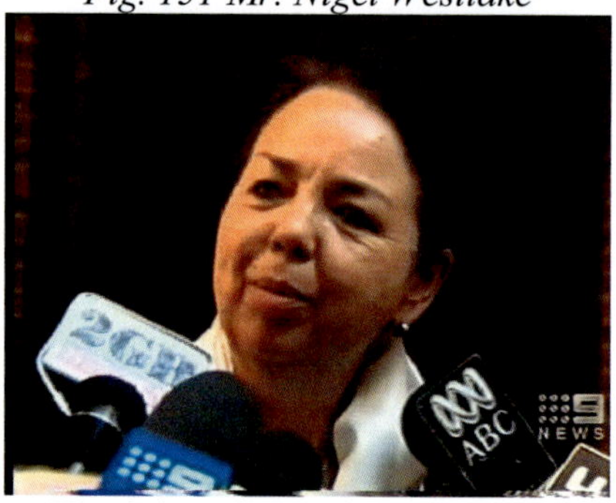

*Fig.152 Mrs. Janice Westlake. Eli Westlake's father and mother, at a news conference after the verdict.*
*[Source: Channel 9 News, Sydney]*

Mr Nigel Westlake concluded that, "The Crown revealed that Eli's life was taken by a complete stranger in a savage act of brutal violence. An act laden with evil intent. An act that can only be described as disturbingly predatory in nature."

A young life snuffed out. In a "senseless act of anger."

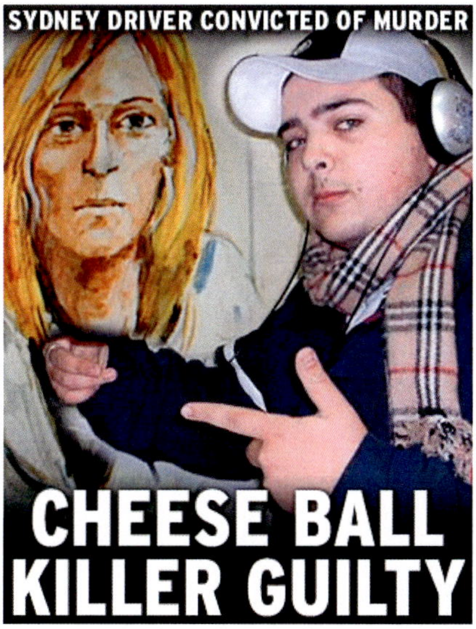


*Fig. 153. This headline appeared in the 'Daily Telegraph' after the verdict was reached with a 'ghostly' cut-&-paste picture of Eli Westlake. [Source: "Daily Telegraph"]*

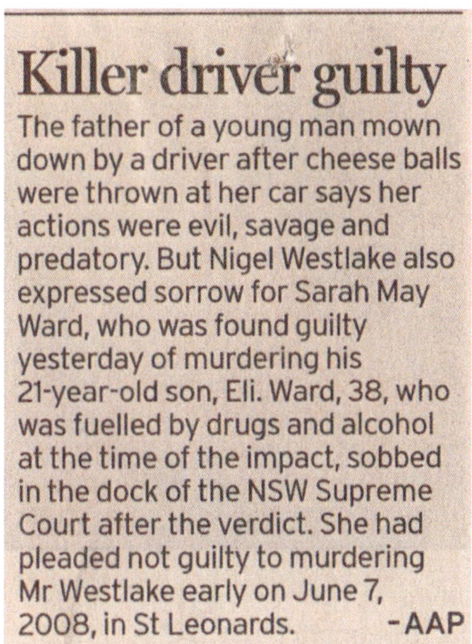

Killer driver guilty

The father of a young man mown down by a driver after cheese balls were thrown at her car says her actions were evil, savage and predatory. But Nigel Westlake also expressed sorrow for Sarah May Ward, who was found guilty yesterday of murdering his 21-year-old son, Eli. Ward, 38, who was fuelled by drugs and alcohol at the time of the impact, sobbed in the dock of the NSW Supreme Court after the verdict. She had pleaded not guilty to murdering Mr Westlake early on June 7, 2008, in St Leonards. -AAP

*Fig. 154. This paragraph also appeared in the 'Sydney Morning Herald' after the verdict was reached.*

# 18
# Dr Suresh Nair – Cocaine Killer

*"Drug misuse is not a disease, it is a decision, like the decision to step out in front of a moving car. You would call that not an error of judgement."*

Phillip K. Dick

**A "Sex Rash" Emerges in the Making of a Surgeon.**

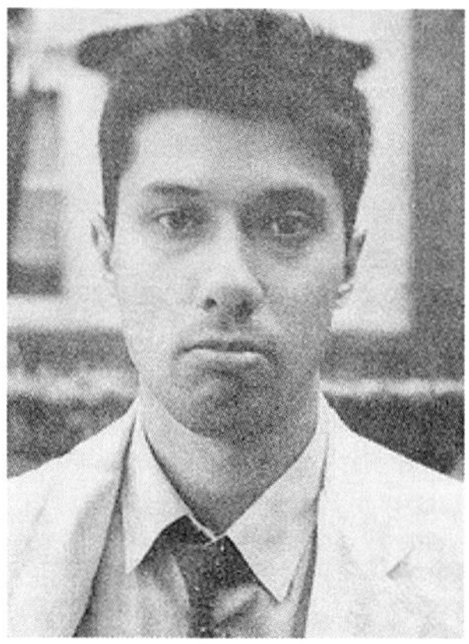

*Fig. 155. Suresh Surendranath Nair's 1991* Sydney University Yearbook *photograph.*

Suresh Surendranath Nair was born in Malaysia to Indian parents who migrated to Australia when Suresh was just ten years of age. They returned home a decade later, leaving Suresh to pursue a medical degree at the University of Sydney. A number of his fellow students remembered him as a very polite, quiet student. Medical training is a demanding experience with the undergraduate studies lasting from five to six years. However, he did have a grubby sense of humour and a liking for pornography, leading to comments to be entered beside his yearbook photograph under the title, 'good points':

"Well, he has a good sense of humour, albeit disgusting. When you think of Suresh Nair, you almost immediately think of grunting and unintelligible mumbling; primeval noises." And "Give him a good *Penthouse* and he's happy."

Some rather prophetic classmates even predicted that by 2011 he would be, "Deregistered and exiled to the rainforests of the Amazon to live with cannibals."

Unfortunately, as events unfolded they were half right. But, who knows about the second!

## The Cocaine Cometh

Suresh was apparently never an outstanding student at Sydney University but even so, he was able to make the necessary grades in medical school before completing his residency and then embarked on surgical training, specialising in neurosurgery. The postgraduate component then involved very long hours as an intern, with life and death decisions to be made on patients. For the most part, Suresh Nair appeared to be a competent doctor and successfully completed his training requirements.

However, it is an unfortunate trait of humans to resort to substance abuse to relieve stress from overwork and/or poor relationships: sexual or otherwise.

Apparently, Dr Nair had both. It was during his postgraduate training that the first signs of his weakness for drugs, cocaine in particular, became evident. A prominent brain surgeon and friend, Dr Charles Teo defended him by saying, “Suresh didn’t have a balanced life, no social life. He was very awkward with girls and in my opinion it seemed like he could not relate to women.”[1]

However, due to his strange behaviour towards his patients and evidence of drug usage, Dr Nair was suspended in 2004, and again in 2008, after which he was forced to undergo regular urine tests and work under supervision. Clearly, cocaine and/or substance abuse was playing an important part in his life. The second suspension related to his clinical practice. But there were more serious problems. Dr Patrick Cregan, a general surgeon and head of quality assurance at Nepean Hospital, said to the Health Care Complaints Commission (HCCC),

“There are significant holes in the concept of supervised practice.It is a myth that you can supervise someone doing surgery.”

This indecision, without any other firm guidelines, led to further serious problems. Sadly, Dr Suresh Nair continued to practice surgery whilst under the likely influence of cocaine and possibly, other stimulants. Despite staff concerns, Dr Nair was allowed to work under ‘supervision’ at the Nepean Hospital. This decision led to unfortunate untoward consequences, resulting in a number of botched operations and, ultimately, the deaths of two young women.

## Botched Operations

We will probably never know how many operations that Dr Nair presided over from 2004 onwards that may have been less than adequate. Only his colleagues would be able to give an estimate to this. However, this is unlikely given the focus upon maintaining a doctor in practice where possible and delaying the necessary disciplinary measures. There now appears to be a long list of patients that will never recover from what was done to them. However, two cases stand out: namely those concerning Ms Helen Kerner and Mrs Debbie Burns.

Helen Kerner had trusted her "nice, clean-cut" neurosurgeon when he said he had performed the delicate spinal operation she required many times before. The sixty-year-old lady was confused when she woke up incontinent of all things, and still in pain, with no feeling in her legs or pelvis, and upset when he tried to discharge her from hospital two days into recovery.

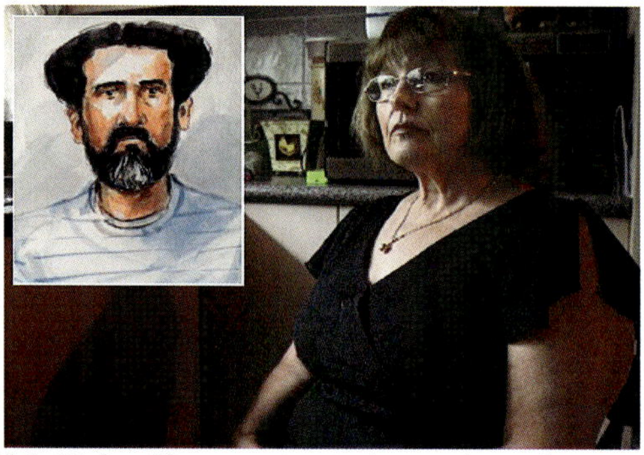

*Fig. 156. Helen Kerner - incontinent since the operation.*
*[Inset, an early court drawing of Suresh Nair.]*
*Picture: Dean Sewell,* Sydney Morning Herald

But when then Dr Suresh Surendranath Nair confessed that his "drill slipped" during the procedure, severing several nerves in her spine, Ms Kerner said she felt sorry for the doctor, who was then thirty-eight. A very forgiving lady.

"I felt like 'my goodness me, he must be feeling awful for what he's done'," Ms Kerner said. "But not now, not now, I'm pretty angry now."

Sydney West Area Health Service has since admitted a breach of duty of care in Ms Kerner's case. However, another neurosurgeon described the procedure, performed in 2006, as a standard operation and said Dr Nair's blunder was "usually so rare as to be virtually unheard of". Previously, after an appearance before the NSW Medical Board's Impaired Registrants Panel in 2004 his surgeon's registration was suspended. He was suspended again in 2008 and again on November 26, 2009.

Ms Kerner, a former relief manager at Anglicare second-hand shops, said she did not know Dr Nair had been suspended when she was referred to him in 2006.

"I had very bad back pain, sciatic pain, and all the doctor had to do was remove a bone spur away from the nerve, just grind it away from the nerve," Ms Kerner continued, "The drill slipped, and my life changed, completely changed."

Ms Kerner was formerly a keen gardener and enjoyed dancing. She now uses walking sticks because she cannot feel her left leg and her foot is deformed. She is bladder and bowel incontinent. In addition, she lost her sexual function and now lives with constant, severe pain in her legs and feet. "I'm very depressed. I wake up in the morning crying sometimes. I'm very embarrassed to go out because of things that happen," she said. "That's my life now. I don't have one."

Ms Kerner said she knew something was wrong when she woke from the anaesthesia, "I spoke to Dr Nair the next morning and he didn't tell me he slipped with the drill. He said he had stretched one of the nerves and it had to be repaired. He said within three months it should heal itself and I believed him because he's my doctor."

Her distress was further compounded when Dr Nair tried to have her discharged from hospital two days after the procedure, before she had been seen by a continence adviser and/or physiotherapist. It was not until Ms Kerner noticed the word *severed* written on her observation chart that she sought answers as to her predicament.

Dr Nair only confessed his blunder when confronted at a meeting with hospital's nursing manager, clinical liaison officer, Ms Kerner and her then partner. After yet another meeting, Ms Kerner was advised by a friend, a continence advisor and two hospital administrators that she could sue for negligence. Legal proceedings began in November 2008 and Sydney West Area Health Services admitted to Ms Kerner's solicitor to a breach of duty of care. Ms Kerner said, "As far as I'm concerned the hospital should have got rid of him at the start, in 2004. If he was gone I wouldn't be like this."

A NSW Supreme Court hearing is to determine what compensation and damages NSW Health must pay Ms Kerner.

Another botched operation concerned Mrs Debbie Burns:

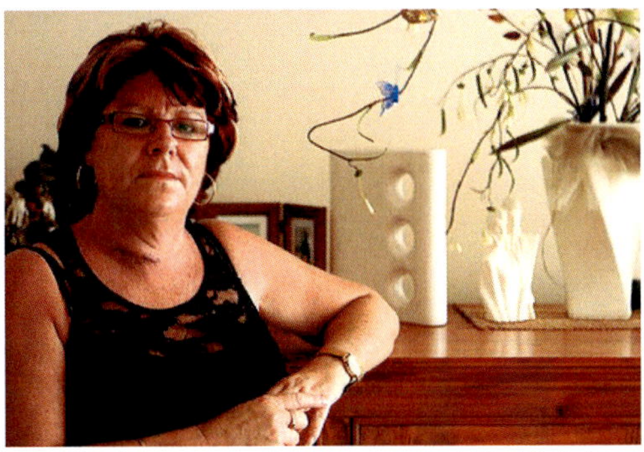

*Fig. 157. Debbie Burns had an operation to correct Dr Nair's surgery on her spine. Photo: Wolter Peeters,* Sydney Morning Herald.

Mrs Debbie Burns, a forty-nine-year-old mother from Werrington, was operated on at Nepean Private Hospital by Dr Suresh Nair for spinal surgery on her neck on October 29, 2010. She was discharged her from hospital Dr Nair over the telephone two days after the surgery that left her unable to hold up her head.

Ms Burns said, "I would do anything to go back to before. The pain that I was experiencing was far worse than the pain before I had the operation."

She further explained that when she woke up from her surgery, she was in extreme pain, with no feeling in her left hand. Dr Nair assured her everything was normal. He put her on morphine and said she should stay in hospital until the following Monday. However, he telephoned her two days later and said he was too unwell to see her and that she could go home. Mrs Burns said she was then discharged with no pain relief medication and woke up the next morning in terrible pain.

"On the Sunday when I got out of bed, it was just terrible. I would stand up for five minutes and have to sit down for twenty minutes to rest my head," she said. "It was excruciating pain. It felt like my head was too heavy for my body."

On November 11, 2010 she was admitted to hospital for "pain management" when her husband, John, complained to Dr Nair's secretary. The family decided to get a second opinion and found out soon afterwards that Dr Nair had been suspended in 2004. He proved to be a very poor choice of a doctor.

Further surgery was clearly necessary to correct the problem. However, she was told by her new surgeon that she may never regain feeling in her left hand.

What these patients did not know was that their surgeon was a cocaine addict, charging thousands of dollars per operation to support his habit. It was a dark secret of a depraved life of cocaine, call girls and all-night orgies.

The Burns family have since filed formal complaints about her care with the NSW Medical Board and the Health Care Complaints Commission.

### The High Life of a Neurosurgeon 'Rock Star'

Initially, Dr Suresh Nair was living a lifestyle that few of us could even dream about. His career as a successful neurosurgeon allowed him the financial freedom to host weekend parties that could rival any rock star's lifestyle.

In some ways, Dr Nair was indeed a 'rock star', only the 'rock' was a potent form of cocaine which he inserted into the bodies of young escorts who came to his luxury $1.7 million Elizabeth Bay apartment in the Eastern Suburbs of Sydney. This sordid practice subsequently resulted in the death of two young women which later proved to be his undoing.

But life outside work was a party and Dr Nair, now in his forties, had the money to pay for it. He also had penchant for lovely looking "model type" girls and desired sex under the influence of drugs, in particular cocaine. He sought high price escorts to satisfy his needs and, consequently, a stream of young women came to his apartment at 15/51 Elizabeth Bay Road, Elizabeth Bay.

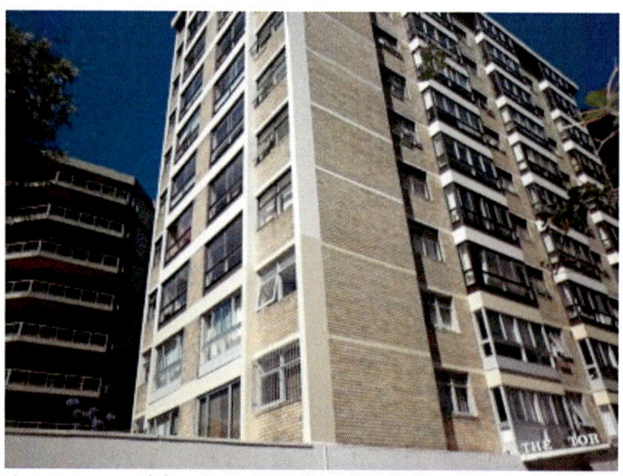

*Fig. 158. Apartment block at 51 Elizabeth Bay Road, Elizabeth Bay.*

Nair was a popular client among Sydney's escorts. A number of the young women came from HM Escorts, Sydney and a number were employed in more 'conventional' jobs ranging from media to banking. The escorts/prostitutes often arrived at his front door apartment and were greeted by Dr Nair offering cocaine lines on a plate. He then urged them to remove their clothing and snort the cocaine before their bacchanalian activities began. These cocaine and sex binges often lasted well into the morning and, as a consequence, began to impact upon his duties as a surgeon and the lives of a number of people associated with him. However, it was mainly due to the tragic deaths of two part-time high class call girls (or escorts) that Dr Suresh Nair's secret depraved life was about to unravel…

**First Casualty: The Death of Victoria McIntyre**

The first of these was that of a pretty young escort (or high class call girl) by the name of Victoria McIntyre, twenty-three years old, who attended one of Dr Nair's fateful cocaine sex 'parties'.

Ms McIntyre worked part-time under the pseudonym of "Lisa" for HM Escorts and she was arranged to visit Dr Nair's residence on February 15, 2009. She was fairly 'new' to the game and used these activities to supplement her regular, more conventional occupation in recruitment management.

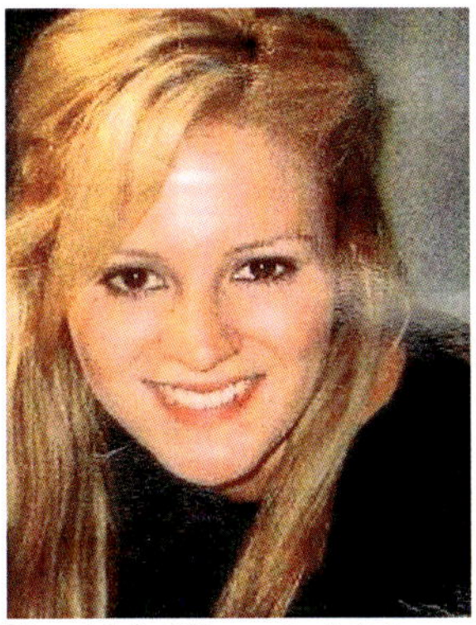

*Fig. 159. Victoria McIntyre*
*Source:* The Daily Telegraph

By the time Ms McIntyre had arrived at the apartment at eleven a.m., drug use and sexual activity had continued throughout the night from one a.m. with two other female escorts, Juliette Lancaster and Elizabeth Carlsen. Another escort had left earlier, after refusing to take the drugs. As Ms McIntyre entered the apartment she was directed by Dr Nair to get naked and take cocaine.

Elizabeth Carlsen warned Ms McIntyre to, "Be wary of the drugs being forced upon you."

She replies, "The only reason I'm here is for the money."

Unfortunately, she did not heed the warning.

Dr Nair then directed the two prostitutes to leave the apartment to go and buy some sex toys and he also writes out a prescription for Xanax. After he hands them the money, they leave the apartment and walk to Kings Cross to carry out their errands.

A short time later, Ms McIntyre began to suffer seizures apparently from the excessive cocaine ingestion. (It was later revealed that 'rocks' of cocaine had been inserted into her anus and vagina. Dr Nair had also directed Ms Lancaster and Ms Carlsen to place some cocaine in their anus. To which Ms Carlsen is said to have complied.) Dr Nair attempted to provide medical support for her seizures and, realising he is unable to help her, contacts an ambulance via the 000 service. In the meantime Ms Lancaster and Ms Carlsen return to the apartment with their purchases, minus the Xanax, and are told by Dr Nair to, 'come back in thirty minutes.'

They then both left via taxi and went to the Sydney Swans AFL club on Darlinghurst Road, Kings Cross and had a drink.

The ambulance attended a short time later to treat the stricken young woman. Ms McIntyre was clearly in a desperate situation as ambulance officers were concerned that she would die and police were contacted. She was then quickly conveyed St Vincent's Hospital where she was incubated and, on examination, emergency staff found her to be brain dead. ("The CT brain scan was recorded as nil focal.") She was immediately placed on life support in the Intensive Care Unit (ICU). When on twelve oh one a.m., Monday 16 February, 2009 it became quite apparent no recovery was possible, and she passed away with family and friends present.

Strangely, Dr Nair, who was suspended previously in 2004 and 2008, was not required to inform the NSW Medical Board of this woman's death in his apartment.

**Second Casualty: The Death of Suellen Dominguez-Zaupa**

The second of these deaths was that of an attractive young escort (or high class call girl) by the name of Suellen Dominguez-Zaupa, twenty-two years old, a Brazilian-born student who attended yet another one of Dr Nair's fateful cocaine sex 'parties'.

Ms Suellen Dominguez-Zauppa was a fun-loving young woman who came from Brazil to study in Sydney, and had the philosophy expressed on Facebook that, "Life looks after those that live it" and had tattooed on her foot, "The World Is Full Of Magic".

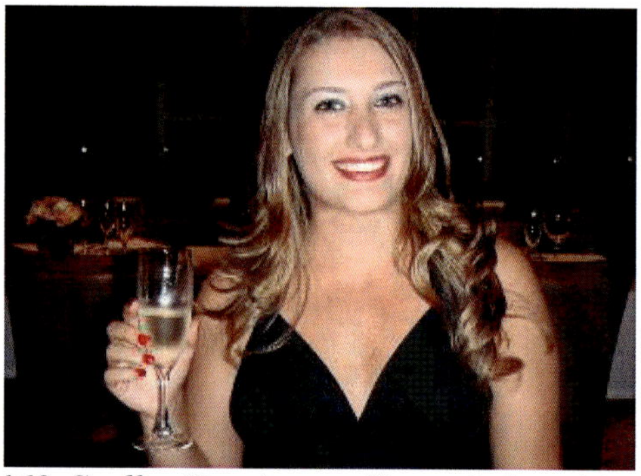

*Fig. 160. Suellen Domingues-Zaupa in happier times.*
*Picture: Facebook*
*Source: The Daily Telegraph*

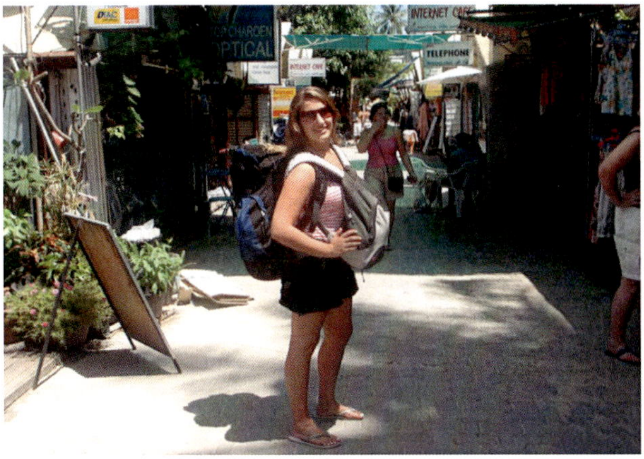

*Fig. 161. Suellen Domingues-Zaupa, 22 in travel mode. [Source: The Daily Telegraph]*

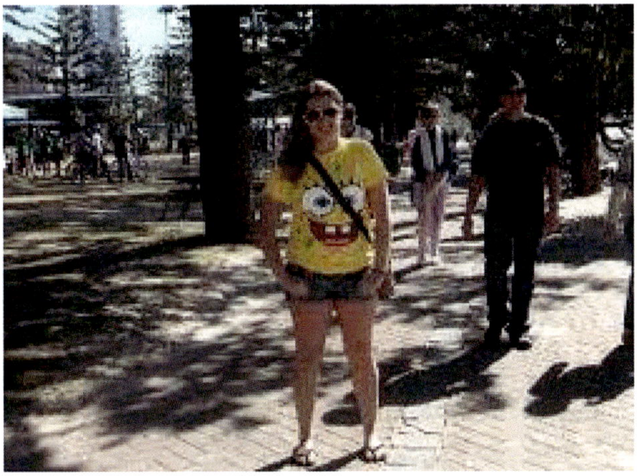

*Festival plans: Suellen Domingues-Zaupa, 22, from Brazil. Picture Source: The Daily Telegraph*

She worked part-time under the pseudonym of 'Nicky' for HM Escorts and she was arranged to visit Dr Nair's residence on November 19, 2009.

Ms Suellen Domingues-Zaupa was also 'new' to the game and apparently used these activities to supplement her studies in hospitality management and travel around Australia. However, these 'extracurricular' activities must have been very discrete as a flatmate commented, "The lifestyle she lived was by no means that of a high-class escort and none of us who knew her well believed she would be capable of doing such a thing."

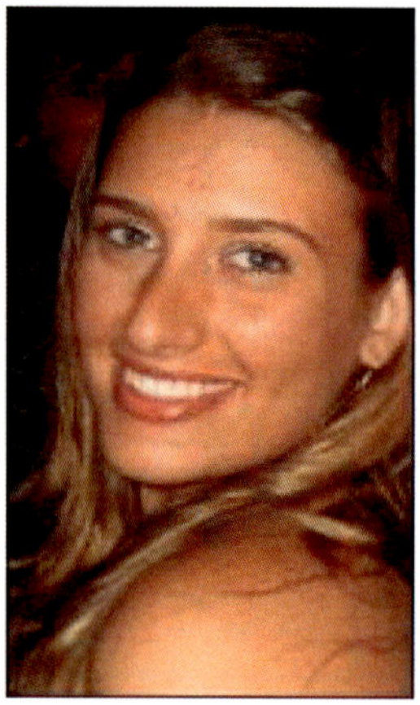

*Fig. 162. Suellen Dominguez-Zaupa*
*Source:* The Age*, 2009*

On the afternoon of November 19, Colombian-born escort, Ms Carmen Hernandez-Cardona ('Catty') arrived at Dr Nair's apartment and received payment from him for four hours' work. He paid by cheque valued at $3200.

She then snorted half a line of cocaine with a fifty-dollar note.

Suellen Domingues-Zaupa or ('Nicky') arrived a short time later and was also given a cheque. They undressed and started, "kissing and cuddling", while taking cocaine, then taking part in an almost four-hour, threesome sex binge.

As she was about to leave as the four hours were coming to an end, she was given a further cheque to stay on. By this time, Ms Domingues-Zauppa began to shake uncontrollably and was having trouble breathing, while 'talking crazy',

"I got bananas in my eyes..." She was not joking.

After about fifteen to twenty minutes her face started to go a grey-blue colour, and bloody saliva was emerging from her mouth. This was a very bad sign, indicating that her bodily functions were shutting down.

Ms Hernandez-Cardona pleaded with Dr Nair to, "Please, do something."

He then allegedly replied, "She'll be all right, I'm a doctor, trust me."

This trust was again misplaced.

When it was apparent that Ms Domingues-Zauppa was dead, he allegedly offered Ms Hernandez-Cardona $50,000 "not to talk to anyone".

She refused the offer and left the apartment.

Meanwhile, back at the Nepean Hospital, staff became concerned that Dr Suresh Nair had not appeared to carry out his duties for the past two days.

Hospital staff contacted Kings Cross Police expressing their concerns. At about seven thirty p.m. on 20 November, 2009 a patrol car was sent to his address in Elizabeth Bay. No persons appeared to be at the address, and so a business card was left under the door requesting contact. No reply was received, and at about two thirty p.m. on Saturday 21 November police returned to the premises and were again unable to gain access. This time entry was forced, and an unpleasant sight befell them. Ms Domingues-Zaupa was found lying face up on a bed in the main bedroom. She had been covered with a "quilt, a towel and two pillows placed intentionally over her head." Her legs were exposed beyond the quilt and she was only wearing underpants. It was clear she had been dead for some time.

Detectives and crime scene officers were notified. Crime scene examination observed that the deceased had froth in her mouth, and she was clutching a new condom in her left hand which had been removed from a packet. There were numerous condoms strewn around the apartment, both opened and unopened, used and unused. Numerous glasses along with empty bottles of vodka were also found. Abundant quantities of white powder were found throughout the apartment. The night had been quite a bacchanalian event.

It was later learned that several other escorts had been entertained in the apartment while Ms Domingues-Zaupa's lifeless body lay in his bed.

Dr Nair was charged on 25 November with supplying drugs in relation to her death, and was also immediately suspended by the NSW Medical Board for the *third time.*

**Post Mortem Examinations of Victims**

Blood samples taken from Victoria McIntyre at the post mortem showed the following results: benzoylecgonine 7.0 milligrams per litre, and cocaine 7.1 milligrams per litre. Cocaine was detected in her nasal and rectal swabs.

Whilst, her post mortem examination, in part, "showed a focal haemorrhagic area in the heart. The lungs were congested and oedematous (abnormal amount of watery fluid present). There were minor injuries to the anal and rectal area and some contusions in the bladder and an abrasion in the rectum.

"Toxicological examination showed toxic levels of cocaine and its metabolite in the blood. Both the nasal and rectal swabs detected cocaine."

The forensic pathologist, Dr R. Janse Van Vuuren concluded, "Based on my examination, both with the naked eye and microscopically, and on evaluation of the neuropathology and toxicology reports, the cause of death in my opinion is acute cocaine toxicity. The findings of acute haemorrhage in the heart, with focal haemorrhage in the brain, in conjunction with the high cocaine levels, are consistent with acute cocaine toxicity."

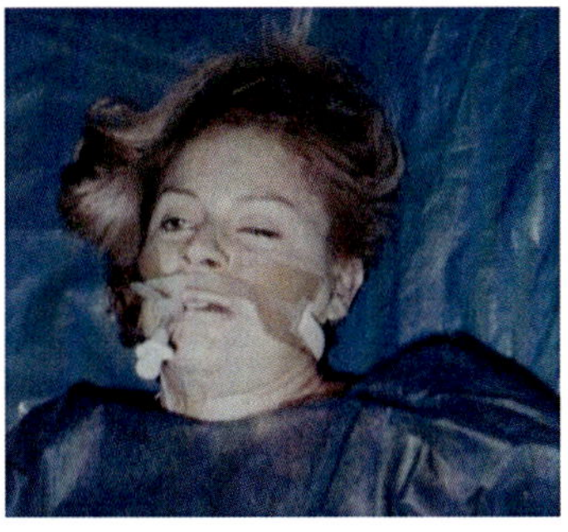

*Fig. 163. Even in death, Victoria McIntyre was a beautiful young woman - a tragic loss.*

I concluded in my report that, "the extremely high level of cocaine detected in Ms McIntyre's blood would have most certainly led to her death."

A blood sample taken from Suellen Domingues-Zaupa at post mortem showed the following results: benzoylecgonine 3.4 milligrams per litre, cocaine 4.9 milligrams per litre, alprazolam (Xanax) 0.009 milligrams per litre, lignocaine at 2 milligrams per litre and delta-9-tetrahydrocannabinol acid (an inactive metabolite of cannabis) 0.017 milligrams per litre. Cocaine, levamisole and lignocaine (the latter two drugs are used as 'cutting' agents for cocaine) were detected in her nasal and rectal swabs.

Whilst, her post mortem examination by Dr Issabella G. Brouwer showed in part, that: "The body was in an early state of decomposition

"The internal organs were in an early state of decomposition and had an autolytic appearance. Both lungs had a mottled appearance.

"Toxicological screening and quantification of blood and other specimens retained at autopsy showed the following:

- Blood preserved contained 4.9 mg/L cocaine. Cocaine concentrations in fatalities range from 0.9-21 mg/L (average 5.3 mg/L). (Baselt, RC. Disposition of Toxic Drugs and Chemicals in Man, Eight Edition, Biomedical Publications, Foster City, California, 2008 p 351).
- The concentration of cocaine detected in the blood of the deceased is therefore consistent with cocaine toxicity.
- 3.4 mg/L of Benzoylecgonine which is a metabolite of cocaine.
- Blood contained 0.009 mg/L (or 9 ug/L) of alprazolam (Xanax). In seven cases of apparent suicide of adults by alprazolam ingestion, the post-mortem blood concentration was 122-2100 ug/L (average 550 ug/L). The concentration of alprazolam detected in the blood of the deceased is therefore well below the toxic levels.
- Delta-9-THC Acid is a metabolite of marijuana (Cannabis sativa).
- Low, non-toxic levels of lignocaine (2 mg/L) were detected. Lignocaine is often used as a cutting agent with cocaine.
- Levamisole has been recorded to be used as a cutting agent with cocaine."

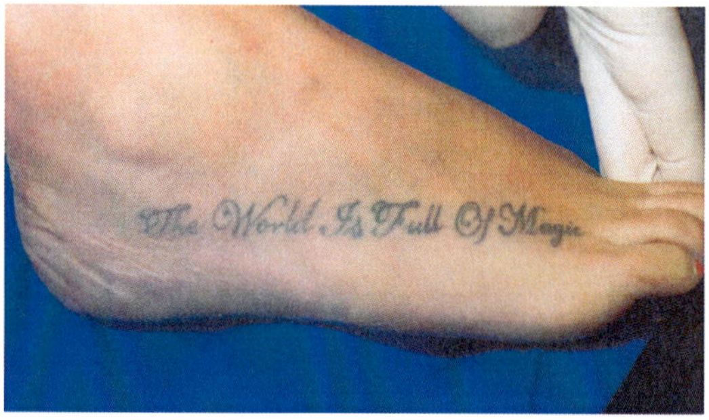


*Fig. 164. A post-mortem picture of Suellen Domingues-Zaupa's foot showing her optimistic tattoo.*

I concluded in my report that, "the toxic level of cocaine detected in (Ms) Domingues-Zaupa's blood would have most certainly led to her death. I am unable to comment on the level of levamisole as this drug was not quantitated. However, the ingestion of levamisole is potentially dangerous and should only be administered under medical supervision."

This appeared to be in agreement with the pathologists' reports and other expert statements. Both victims had died through the excessive ingestion of cocaine.

## Called to Account

Suresh Surendranath Nair was treated very fairly under the Australian justice system and possibly excessively fair by the Medical Board given the number of suspensions he received for his nefarious activities, to the detriment of his patients.

He was eventually charged with causing the death of Victoria McIntyre, in circumstances amounting to manslaughter. He was also charged with murdering Suellen Domingues-Zaupa and the supply of a prohibited drug on both occasions. However, he was originally granted bail provided he did not hire any sex workers or took prohibited drugs.

Cocaine and sex can prove to be a powerful combination, and in this case, impossible to resist. Suresh Nair was arrested on 9 January, 2010 shortly after midnight, when Kings Cross detectives raided his rented apartment in Hall Street, Bondi. When officers knocked on his door, he answered and allegedly called out to the women in the bedroom:

"Girls put your clothes on. The police are here. It's over."

His arrest came after surveillance police alleged that he separately hired three female escorts between nine thirty p.m. and eleven fifteen p.m. and, taking them back to the first floor Bondi apartment, allegedly partook in cocaine with two of the escorts. The police raid on the apartment came a week after Dr Nair had discharged himself from a private hospital, where he had been undergoing treatment for his addictions as part of his bail conditions.

The leniency granted to the former Dr Nair was about to end.

In applying for further bail on 11 January, 2010 in Sydney Central Local Court, Nair's solicitor, Mitchell Cavanagh admitted his client had a problem. He told the Court that his client would not reoffend if he was allowed to live with his mother, and would stay at a psychiatric hospital if necessary.

Mr Cavanagh said, "He realises now he cannot trust himself to be on his own."

The application was refused by Magistrate Jane Culver who said that, "This is a matter where the protection of the community looms large. This court can have little confidence in the defendant's willingness to comply with bail conditions."

Mr Nair was taken into custody and taken to Silverwater Gaol.

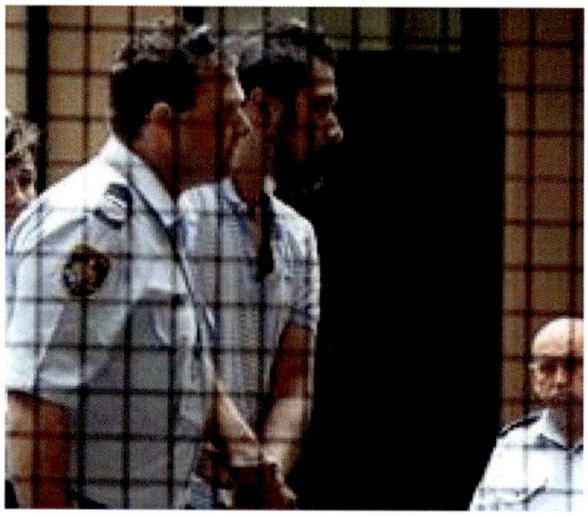

*Fig. 165 'Dr' Suresh Nair being escorted to prison [Source:* The Daily Telegraph*, 2010].*

**Remorse and Regrets**

After some months in gaol, Suresh Nair appeared to have had time to reflect over the events which led up to his present predicament and the destruction of other lives. During this time while in custody, he was assaulted by four inmates where he suffered multiple facial fractures including a broken jaw and broken teeth. Because of the attack he lost partial sight in one eye and was without feeling in his left cheekbone. He was briefly placed in protective custody after the incident.

In a Supreme Court bail hearing on June 25, 2010, Mr Nair's barrister, Peter Hamill SC called psychiatrist Dr Rosalie Wilcox to give evidence about the former surgeon's sex and cocaine addictions. Dr Wilcox said that he had, "more time to think about how his addiction led to the destruction of his life and other lives as well. I believe now that he has been in custody for six months that denial has well and truly confronted."

She continued her expert opinion, "He has come to terms with the seriousness of his addiction and the consequences of his actions."

Mr Nair said that, "I'm really saddened that these two very young girls that died could be caught up in my behaviour.

He was again denied bail, due to the *"strength of his addiction"* and the likelihood that he would reoffend.

In the meantime, the Health Care Complaints Commission (HCCC) was to review all surgery performed at Nepean Public Hospital under the direction of the then Dr Suresh Nair. At the time of writing, that report is yet to surface.

**The Committal Trial**

At a committal hearing for Mr Nair at Sydney's Downing Centre Local Court beginning on December 6, 2010, a number of other witnesses came forward and gave evidence in relation to this matter, including myself. I was amongst the last to give evidence, and was there to interpret the levels of drugs detected in the victim's blood samples.

Mr Nair was accused of two offences: the murder of Brazilian student and escort, Suellen Domingues-Zaupa in November 2009, after she was allegedly supplied with cocaine at his Elizabeth Bay apartment, as well as the manslaughter of fellow escort, Victoria McIntyre in February, 2009.

A number of women with connections to the sex industry, who had been clients of Mr Nair, gave evidence that on arrival at his residence, he would greet them with a plate on which there were lines of cocaine and urge them, " to get coked up."

An interesting aspect of this case was the number of people who led double lives. Several witnesses, all former or current sex workers, included a woman working in the media, a daughter of a chief executive of a major company and a woman working in the banking industry. In addition, for those concerned about the effects on their 'regular' occupations and personal relationships, Crown prosecutor Ms Kate Thompson applied to have the witnesses' names suppressed, saying it would cause damage to their careers and personal relationships if they were outed as former and current sex workers.

The police officers involved in the case, Detective Senior Constables Ben Tearne, Gavin Bradbury and Brad Semken provided testimony about the fears that the eight escort witnesses had about having their identities revealed.

Magistrate Carolyn Barkell rejected the application for all cases except for one woman "Emily" who had since returned to the United States. However, she was subsequently cross-examined via audio-visual link and told the court that she was at Dr Nair's apartment at the time Ms McIntyre overdosed on February 15, 2009. She also said that she told Ms Anna Monaghan, the director of HM International escorts agency that the group were, "taking a lot of drugs and they were putting it into their orifices."

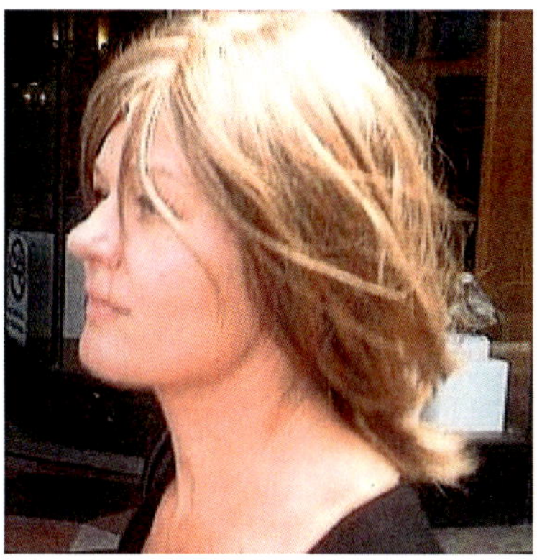

*Fig. 166. Ms Anna Monaghan, director of HM International Escorts*
*[Source:* Sydney Morning Herald
*Photo: Georgina Robinson].*

A medical expert, from Royal Prince Alfred Hospital emergency department, Dr Timothy Green was called to give evidence and told the court that the then Dr Nair, would have recognised the warning signs of cocaine toxicity and should have called an ambulance when Ms Domingues-Zaupa was suffering seizures.

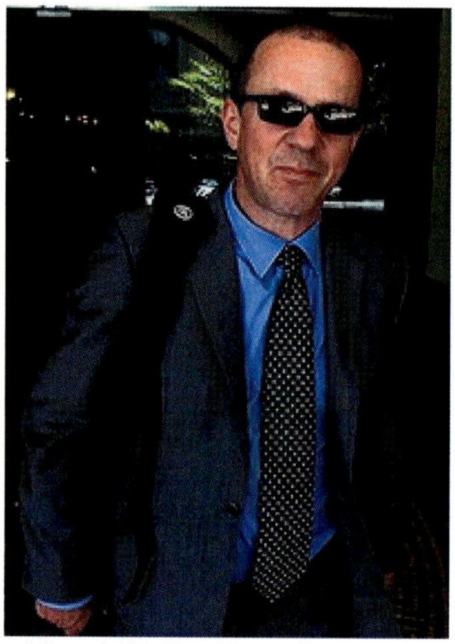

*Fig. 167. Dr Timothy Green*
*Source:* Sydney Morning Herald
*Photo: Dallas Kilponen.*

Dr Green further stated that her seizures, "These seizures could have been successfully treated by a medic", by intravenous medication.

Pathologists, Rianie van Vuuren and Issabella Brouwer, who carried out the post mortems on Ms McIntyre and Ms Domingues-Zaupa respectively, also provided evidence in this matter. Dr Rianie van Vuuren was of the opinion that through the toxicology analysis and in the absence of any other symptoms in her body that she had died from cocaine toxicity.

I was the second last witness to give evidence about Ms McIntyre's and Ms Domingues-Zaupa's deaths at the Downing Centre Local Court.

On attending the court I noticed Mr Nair, in custody, was now clean-shaven and wearing prison greens.

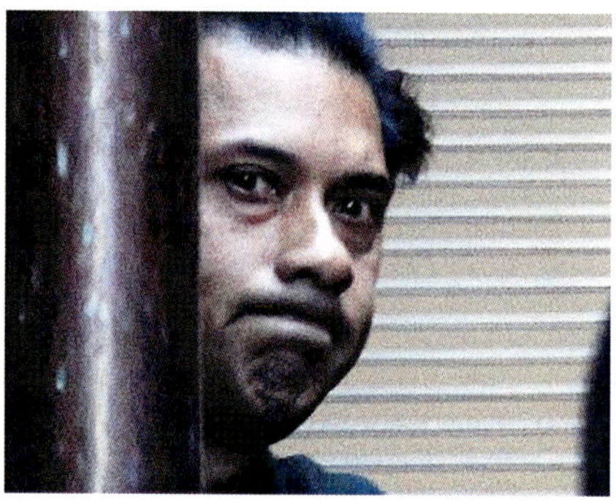

*Fig. 168. A shaven (Mr) Suresh Nair at court.*
*[Source:* Sydney Morning Herald, *December 9, 2010*
*Picture: Nick Moir].*

Mr Peter Hamill SC was Mr Nair's barrister, and I was cross examined on a number of issues relating to cocaine ingestion, including levels of drug found in the victim's blood samples, time of absorption, onset of effects and tolerance.

Whilst the cocaine level in Ms Domingues-Zaupa's blood was very high at 4.9 milligrams per litre of blood and sufficient to cause death, Ms McIntyre's cocaine concentration in her blood of 7.1 milligrams per litre was truly extraordinary.

I told the court, "This is probably one of the highest levels of cocaine I've seen in my career."

Given that I had worked as a forensic scientist for more than thirty-two years, the last ten years with the NSW Police (at the time of writing), this was no overstatement. Also, the administration of cocaine via the anus (and vagina) increased absorption of the drug and allowed it to enter the bloodstream "at a much greater rate," which would account for the extreme cocaine levels detected in the victim's blood.

However, Mr Hamill pursued the issue of Ms McIntyre's medical history, and whether I considered this when making my findings.

He then asked, "Do you agree with the proposition that it is impossible and highly dangerous to speculate on the cause of death from cocaine, based on toxicology alone?"

I replied, "I generally prefer to base my findings on symptoms", and thought the elevated level of cocaine in Ms McIntyre's blood was more than sufficient to cause death, aside from any prior symptoms that may have been observed.

[Note: Cocaine concentrations in some thirty-seven fatalities recorded ranged from 0.04- 31 mg/L (average 4.6 mg/L).Both victims were well over this average level]

The final committal hearing witness was Ms Tanya Verhoeven, who was employed by Sydney Select Escorts at the time of Ms McIntyre's death. She told the court Dr Nair was a popular client with Sydney's escorts.

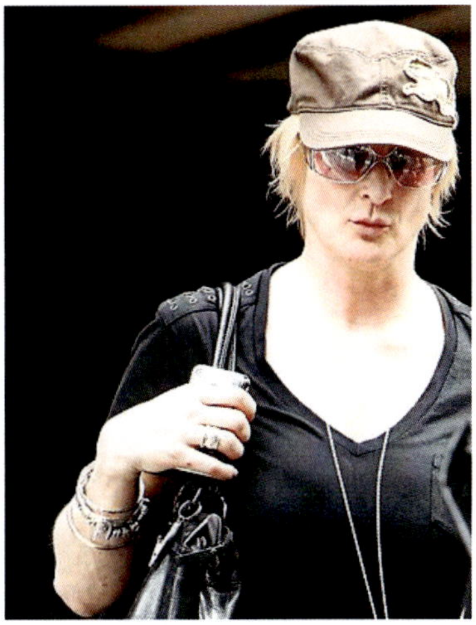

*Fig. 169. Ms Tanya Verhoeven outside court on December 10, 2010 [Source:* Sydney Morning Herald*: Picture: Brad Hunter].*

Ms Verhoeven said that Dr Nair "liked girls who looked like models ... He liked lovely looking girls. A good figure. Not too many curves .... I never before thought he, as a doctor, would ever behave in a dangerous manner."

Ms Verhoeven said she had organised for Ms Juliett Lancaster or 'Jamie' to attend his Valentine's Day "party" at Dr Nair's apartment. She further told the court that Ms Lancaster phoned her on February 15 to tell her that "police cars are everywhere" and that "something had happened."

**Murder Charge Dropped, Manslaughter Charge Maintained**

Suresh Nair subsequently appeared before Judge Robert Toner at Sydney District Court for sentencing on 26 August, 2011.

Mr Nair was initially accused of two offences: the murder of Ms Suellen Domingues-Zaupa in November 2009, as well as the manslaughter of fellow escort, Ms Victoria McIntyre in February, 2009. Both women were allegedly supplied with cocaine at his Elizabeth Bay apartment.

What a wonderful thing plea bargaining is – for the defendant. Both charges were reduced markedly. Suresh Nair pleaded guilty to the manslaughter of Ms Domingues-Zaupa and her murder charge was dropped. He also pleaded guilty to supplying cocaine to Ms McIntyre and her manslaughter charge dropped.

Prior to sentencing Mr Nair, Judge Toner heard complimentary references from former patients of the neurosurgeon, and a glowing testimony from a leading brain surgeon, Dr Charlie Teo.

Judge Toner commented, "It is hard to underestimate the fall of the prisoner.

"I find this evidence powerful and at the same time, difficult to reconcile with the man who committed these crimes, where he essentially abandoned his sense of responsibility.

"Such, though, are the contradictions in this profoundly sad case."

Mr Nair was sentenced to a maximum of nine years gaol, with a non-parole period of five years and four months. As he had been in custody since January 2010, he will be eligible for parole on April 30, 2015.

**Through the 'Cracks' and a very Public Downfall**

Could these tragic events that unfolded have been prevented? Possibly.

Few people get *three* chances to sort out their lives before it impacts upon their career choice, and on other lives in the community. Unfortunately, Dr Nair had 'slipped through cracks in the system' where he was still able to practise medicine, while there was abundant evidence of drug usage some years earlier, before his fall from grace. Several of Dr Nair's colleagues expressed concern about him returning to work after yet another suspension. However, in spite of the concerns, Dr Nair was allowed to return to work albeit, under supervision.

So, who is responsible for an impaired doctor? The Medical Board, the doctor's supervisor and/or employer, or the Health Care Complaints Commission?

In reality, probably all of these bodies, aided by good communication, so that the true nature of a doctor's problems were known.

In the meantime, all surgery performed at Nepean Public Hospital under the direction of the then Dr Suresh Nair is apparently being reviewed. Have lessons been learnt from this case? Hopefully, yes, for all professionals concerned, and better treatment any future patients that may come under the 'care' of an impaired doctor.

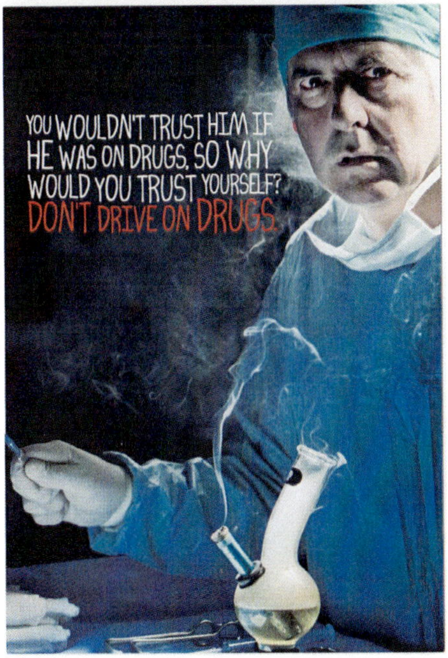
YOU WOULDN'T TRUST HIM IF
HE WAS ON DRUGS, SO WHY
WOULD YOU TRUST YOURSELF?
DON'T DRIVE ON DRUGS.

*Fig. 170 Copy of a brochure handed out at the 2010 ICADTS (International Committee on Alcohol, Drugs and Traffic Safety) Conference held at Oslo, Norway.*

# 19
# Death of a Dancer

*"Dancing faces you towards Heaven, whichever direction you turn."*
Terri Guillemets

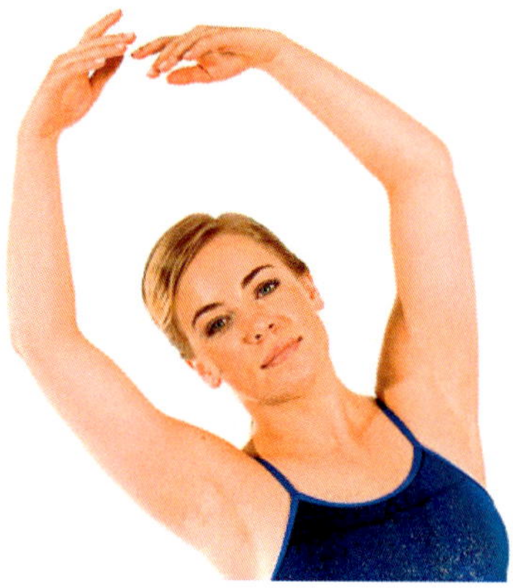

*Fig. 171 Ms Annabel Catt, an accomplished dancer and beautiful human being. Picture courtesy of 2006* Herald and Weekly Times.

**The 'Dark Cousin' – A New Drug on the Block?**

Ecstasy has become a popular drug of abuse.

The drug has no approved medical use in Australia but is widely abused. Injecting has been reported as having the quickest onset and producing a more intense but shorter-lasting experience. The effect of taking larger doses was reported as mainly hallucinatory, an increase that included undesirable side effects as the dose is increased. The onset of action of the drug is usually within thirty to forty minutes and a maximal response is achieved in about one to two hours. The duration of action is about four to six hours (mean five hours) and the drug and its metabolites are excreted, mainly in the urine.

The negative effects of Ecstasy are *dose-related*, in that their severity correlated with both the total number of doses consumed and the *frequency of use.* Short-term high dose use of MDMA has produced incidences of an amphetamine-like psychosis and, in some cases, severe hyperthermia that becomes unresponsive to medical intervention leading to death.

However, these properties are bad enough, without another more deadly 'cousin' drug of MDMA 'lurking in the wings' – this drug is known as para-methoxy-amphetamine or PMA.

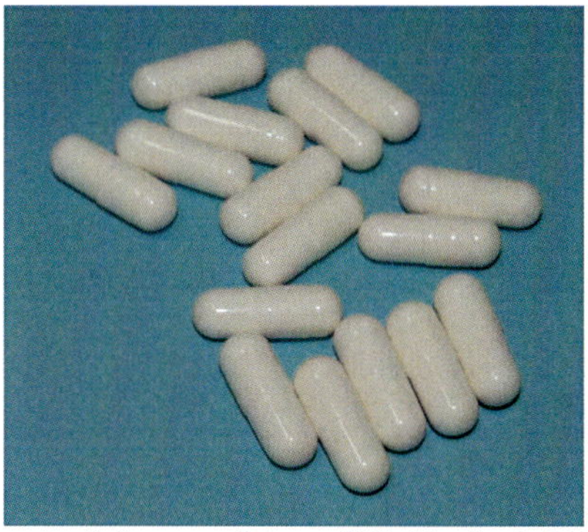

*Fig. 172. A typical dosage form of PMA aka MDMA capsules.*

This drug is one of a group of methoxylated phenethylamine derivatives or so-called 'designer' drugs with marked hallucinogenic properties. PMA has about five times the potency of the naturally occurring drug, mescaline. A number of fatalities from PMA have been reported. Hyperpyrexia (elevated body temperature), agitation ('fitting'), tachycardia (racing heartbeat), shallow laboured breathing and hypertension (elevated blood pressure) are common symptoms of overdosage. PMA is a highly toxic amphetamine drug which is often passed off as Ecstasy and has been linked to a number of deaths in Australia and overseas. The psychoactive effects of PMA have a slower onset than MDMA. PMA is often sold as MDMA and, as such, the increased effects and slower onset can create a very dangerous situation for users, by encouraging consumption of larger quantities of the drug.

This awful drug has managed to infiltrate the 'drug scene' mostly because it was easier to get than the precursor chemicals for the synthesis of 3, 4-methylenedioxymethamphetamine. This 'cheapened' drug was about to impact adversely on another innocent life…

**A 'Bubbly' Dancer**

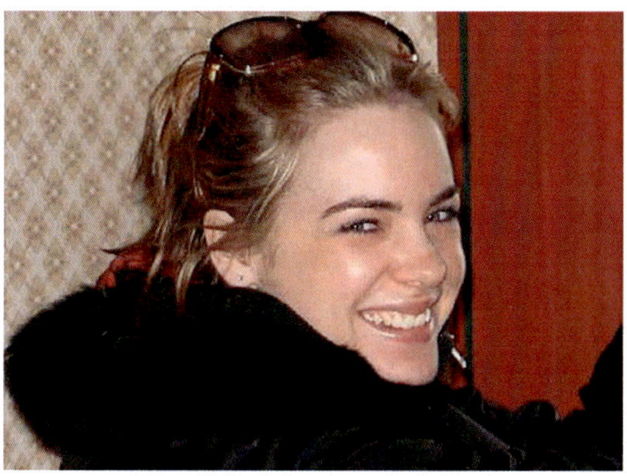

*Fig. 173. Ms. Annabel Catt.*
*Photograph: Courtesy Channel Seven.*

With her infectious smile and cheeky nature, Annabel Catt could get away with almost anything. As her brother Anthony recalled, "She could get away with almost anything and persuade almost anyone with a special combination *of straight honesty and a cheeky smile on her face."*

Annabel's true passion was dancing and was a part-time dance teacher at an Avalon dance school and had been at Brent Street performing arts school since 2001. Dancing was an important part of her life. Even when she played basketball or netball, "She danced across the court," said her mother Alison.

But at the Good Vibrations music festival, she was about to test her luck once too many times. The combination of the drugs, MDMA and PMA – in particular – was to lead to a tragic death of a beautiful talented twenty-year-old Australian woman, a dancer, dance teacher and former vice-captain of Narrabeen Sports High School...

**The Good Vibrations Festival, Sydney**

It seems prior to this incident that she had attended the Good Vibrations Festival (or 'GVF') on the 17 February, 2007. It was a very warm and sunny day and everyone appeared to be in a good spirits, keen to listen and dance to some top musical acts. The GVF began in 2003, and has now become a landmark on the Australian summer calendar. Its travelling circus consists of a variety of acts including the Beastie Boys, Timo Maas, Nightmares On Wax, Jurassic 5, Cassius, Rhazel, JS-one, Thunderball, DJ Yoda and Fort Knox Five along with a variety of other acts.

In Sydney Centennial Park the GVF drew a crowd of 32,000 music fans who sweated to the sounds of the above, joined by DJ Dan, Cut Copy, Cicada, Ursula 1000 and Kraak & Smaak.

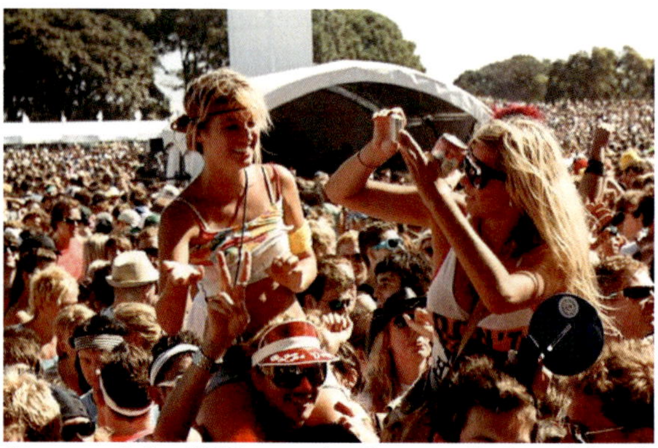

*Fig. 174. Picture of the GVF crowd – Source:* Sydney Morning Herald.

It was apparently a "smashing success" with special guests such as Snoop Dog and the Beastie Boys "stealing the show". A popular venue for young folk. Unfortunately also for drug dealers who saw it as a 'candy shop' for revellers looking to buy drugs...

## A Fateful Day

It started out as a regular fun weekend music festival, mixing it with friends, and having a good time. Annabelle just loved the music, the new bands – and the dancing. At about two p.m., as the music blared out from the festival in Sydney's Centennial Park, Annabel and a group of her friends sat down on the grass to enjoy the music – and a tablet or two of Ecstasy. However, this day was going to be quite different for Annabel.

Annabel's friend, Bodene Sheed in the meantime had collected from her boyfriend six Ecstasy tablets and six capsules of MDMA. The latter supposedly a powder form of Ecstasy. The plastic bag containing the drugs was passed around. A deadly drug combination situation was about to unfold.

Around four p.m. that afternoon, Annabel Catt and one of her friends, Danielle Lettoof took another Ecstasy tablet. Then, with the effects of the first tablet wearing off, both decided to take a MDMA capsule. After initially feeling no reaction, Annabel then took a second capsule sometime later, as they headed for home. Those capsules contained PMA, a killer-in-waiting. As they travelled home on the bus, they were hallucinating, sweating and unable to walk properly. Annabel was starting to experience further adverse effects of the drugs and was knocking the seat in front of her as her leg muscles went into spasms.

Her arms tightened and veins popped out. On reaching Mona Vale, Annabel was helped into her home suffering from hyperthermia. As her temperature was so high, a shower should do the trick. Not a problem. She was a bit agitated, but so were the other girls. Well, off to bed. During the night Annabelle was suffering, and the spasms in her legs appeared to have worsened causing her to kick a chest of drawers at the foot of her bed. The noise woke her companions, who turned on the light and realised that she was having some difficulty in breathing and she had turned an "eerie ice blue." Her friend, Danielle Lettoof showed similar symptoms but was not as severely affected. However, her eyes were extremely dilated and she was also exhibiting physical signs of hyperthermia. At this point Danielle would have had no idea how much she, too, was in danger. An ambulance was called and the two young women were rushed off to Mona Vale Hospital arriving at the Intensive Care Unit in just eight minutes at five thirty a.m. Annabelle's body temperature was 41.9 degrees Celsius – a dangerously high temperature, given the body's normal temperature is 37.5 degrees Celsius. An ice bag was applied to lower her temperature and she was intubated.

Danielle had not taken the other deadly capsule, as she had become physically ill about an hour later after taking the first MDMA capsule, and had warned the others not to take theirs because of her reaction. [The remaining capsule was later handed to the Police to have it analysed.] However, the drugs were affecting Danielle as she was pale, her eyes "extremely dilated" and was showing physical signs of hyperthermia. But she was still lucid, and able to inform police that she and Annabel had taken an "MDMA cap" each, which had been purchased from Bodene Sheed. Bodene in turn had obtained the "caps" from her boyfriend prior to attending the Good Vibrations Festival.

In the meantime, Medical staff was taking heroic efforts to save Annabelle's life. They administered midazolam to reduce the seizures and spasms, they gave her electric shocks to get her heart back into rhythm and she was ventilated to aid her breathing. But it was a losing battle. The outcome may have been quite different had she reached hospital sooner, – much sooner.

A much beloved 'bubbly' dancer, Annabel Jane Catt passed away at six thirteen a.m., a terrible loss. Her friend, Danielle Lettoof, fortunately survived the ordeal.

## Blood Levels Found

A blood sample taken from Annabelle Catt at the autopsy was found to contain MDMA at 0.5 milligrams per litre, midazolam less than 0.1 milligrams per litre and 4-methoxyamphetamine (or para-methoxyamphetamine, or PMA) 1.9 milligrams per litre.

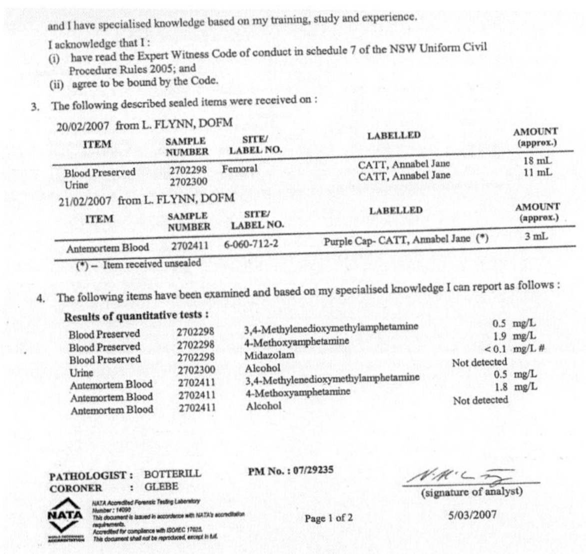

and I have specialised knowledge based on my training, study and experience.

I acknowledge that I :
(i) have read the Expert Witness Code of conduct in schedule 7 of the NSW Uniform Civil Procedure Rules 2005; and
(ii) agree to be bound by the Code.

3. The following described sealed items were received on :

20/02/2007 from L. FLYNN, DOFM

| ITEM | SAMPLE NUMBER | SITE/ LABEL NO. | LABELLED | AMOUNT (approx.) |
|---|---|---|---|---|
| Blood Preserved | 2702298 | Femoral | CATT, Annabel Jane | 18 mL |
| Urine | 2702300 | | CATT, Annabel Jane | 11 mL |

21/02/2007 from L. FLYNN, DOFM

| ITEM | SAMPLE NUMBER | SITE/ LABEL NO. | LABELLED | AMOUNT (approx.) |
|---|---|---|---|---|
| Antemortem Blood | 2702411 | 6-060-712-2 | Purple Cap- CATT, Annabel Jane (*) | 3 mL |

(*) – Item received unsealed

4. The following items have been examined and based on my specialised knowledge I can report as follows :

**Results of quantitative tests :**

| | | | |
|---|---|---|---|
| Blood Preserved | 2702298 | 3,4-Methylenedioxymethylamphetamine | 0.5 mg/L |
| Blood Preserved | 2702298 | 4-Methoxyamphetamine | 1.9 mg/L |
| Blood Preserved | 2702298 | Midazolam | < 0.1 mg/L # |
| Urine | 2702300 | Alcohol | Not detected |
| Antemortem Blood | 2702411 | 3,4-Methylenedioxymethylamphetamine | 0.5 mg/L |
| Antemortem Blood | 2702411 | 4-Methoxyamphetamine | 1.8 mg/L |
| Antemortem Blood | 2702411 | Alcohol | Not detected |

PATHOLOGIST : BOTTERILL
CORONER : GLEBE

PM No. : 07/29235

(signature of analyst)

NATA Accredited Forensic Testing Laboratory
Number: 14090
This document is issued in accordance with NATA's accreditation requirements.
Accredited for compliance with ISO/IEC 17025.
This document shall not be reproduced, except in full.

Page 1 of 2

5/03/2007

*Fig. 175. The Analyst's Report*
*[Division of Analytical Laboratories, Lidcombe, NSW].*

I found the level of MDMA in her blood was particularly high given the therapeutic range is 0.1-0.35 milligrams per litre for the 'feel good' euphoria effects, etc, sought by users of the drug, which indicated several tablets had been taken. But, more importantly, so was the level of PMA which was well within the lethal range. This indicated a very high dosage. The remaining capsule given to the police officer was analysed and found to contain a very high content of PMA at 44.5%. As I indicated in my subsequent statement: "the level of PMA in Ms CATT's blood would have been more than sufficient to result in her death, even without the additive effects from MDMA."

## The Aftermath

The popular dancer's death struck a deep chord with the community. Grief counselling was provided to her friends who were with Annabel. All were encouraged to seek ongoing trauma/grief counselling.

On February 21, 2007 Bodene Sheed of Mona Vale was charged at Dee Why police station with supplying a prohibited drug namely, PMA and Ecstasy at the Good Vibrations Festival. She was granted conditional bail to appear at Manly Local Court on 21 March 2007. The matter was subsequently moved to the Downing Centre Local Court, where Bodene Sheed appeared before Magistrate Robert Williams for sentencing.

Members of the Catt family were not present.

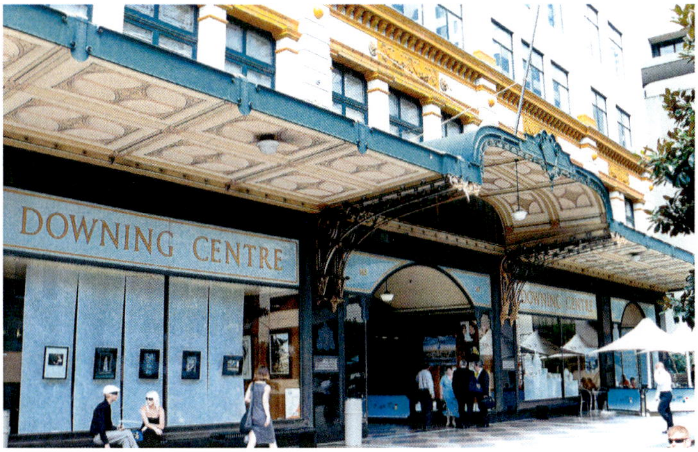


*Fig. 176. Sydney's Downing Centre Courts*

Ms Bodene Sheed pleaded guilty to two counts of supplying a prohibited drug namely, six tablets of Ecstasy and six MDMA capsules.

In an opening address, his honour said it was clear the offence had a tragic result that Ms Sheed may not have been able to foresee.

"But the difficulty in this matter is that that is what happened," as he continued, "There possibly could not have been a more tragic result, but I am sure this has been brought home to you."

Ms Sheed's barrister, Mr Anthony Jamieson, described his client as "deeply remorseful" and said she made no money from the supply, merely passing on the bag of tablets which were obtained from another person. In addition, he said:

"All of the girls had freely been using drugs."

His Honour Williams noted Ms Sheed's remorse and the fact that the drug supply was not a large one, but still it played a significant part in the tragedy.

"Even though the evidence and statements indicate that the users or persons to whom you supplied the drugs on this night were persons who had used drugs on prior occasions," he said, "Notwithstanding that, a message must be sent to the community that Parliament and also the courts are against the supply of drugs in any quantity."

He continued, "I must also recognise the harm done to the victim, in this case the ultimate harm, and to the community," he said.

Detective Sergeant Stephen Pollard, who investigated the case, told the magistrate that there had been no other arrests in relation to the matter. He said that the defendant had been "very forthcoming, and that the information she had given him was to the best of her knowledge."

Magistrate Robert Williams said although she could not have known the tragic consequences that would unfold, she still had to take responsibility for her actions. He then sentenced her to 120 hours of community service.

Ms Sheed shed tears in the box, and nodded as Magistrate Williams warned another slip up would leave her in jail.

Outside Downing Centre court, Ms Sheed was asked by reporters was she remorseful over her friend's death, and that she would never use drugs again.

To which she replied, "Yes" to each question, before being driven hurriedly away.

**Lessons Learned?**

Mrs Alison Catt, the deceased's mother, somewhat generously, told ABC radio that she believed Ms Bodene Sheed was also a victim.

"We see her as another victim really," she said, "She was the foot soldier in this and we're glad she has been able to help the police with further investigations." She continued, "I think why it's been reported so widely is because we are an ordinary family and she was just a fun-loving, ordinary girl and she wasn't into drugs, so this can happen to anyone."

Mrs Catt concluded that she hoped lessons would be learnt from her daughter's death.

Annabel Catt's father, Peter said, "We really wish that if anything positive comes out of the loss of our dear Annabel, it is that other people would think twice before taking any kind of drug."

**Conclusion**

The question as to why Annabel Catt died while her companion, Danielle Lettooff survived has been considered. The answer lies in the dosages of the drugs taken. It was believed that Ms Lettoof had taken the first capsule earlier in the afternoon than did Ms Catt, and that later both took their remaining capsules at the same time. This may have contributed to Ms Lettoof's reaction to the drug that, while serious, was not fatal. In fact, the other capsule had not been ingested by Ms Lettoof and was handed to a police officer.

[An analysis of a blood sample taken at the hospital would have shed some light on this outcome.]

The post-mortem blood levels obtained from Annabel Catt for either drug were at lethal proportions, in particular the PMA but including the MDMA, and sadly a fatal outcome was pretty much inevitable despite medical intervention. Had Danielle Lettoof consumed that other capsule containing the PMA, the final outcome would have been, most likely even more tragic: with the deaths of *two* young people.

# 20
# The Antique Knife

*"First you take a drink, then the drink takes a drink,*
*then the drink takes you."*

F. Scott Fitzgerald

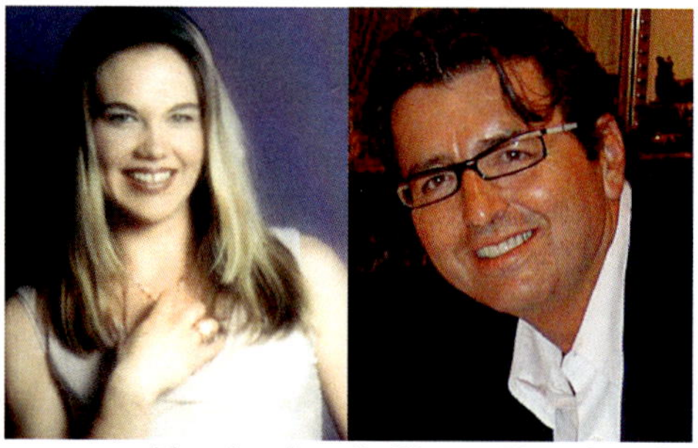

*Fig. 177 Danielle Stewart and her husband, Chaim Kimel, in happier times. Pictures courtesy of Sydney* Morning Herald.

## Prequel

When Chiam Kimel met Danielle Stewart at a Kings Cross nightclub, he would not have known how his relationship with the slight pretty woman, about half his age at the time, and the purchase of a decorative antique knife on a holiday with her, would affect his life – and ultimately, his death.

Chiam Kimel (fifty-five years old) had been in a relationship with Danielle Stewart (thirty years old) for about six years, and they had been married for the previous three of those years. Unfortunately, for the couple these latter years were not easy, as Danielle suffered from a history of mental illness and self-harming, which led to various domestic issues and screaming matches. Chiam and Danielle resided together in rented accommodation in unit number 18/740 New South Head Road, Rose Bay. This unit had two bedrooms on the fourth level of the residential complex. The couple shared shared the unit with Jordan Kimel, a sixteen year old, the son of Chiam Kimel, from a previous relationship.

## A Pleasant Dinner with Friends

On the evening of the 23 August 2006 Danielle Stewart and Chiam Kimel went to dinner with friends, Angela Batley and Harley Nash, at the Pescator Fish and Grill Restaurant on New South Head Road at Rose Bay. On arriving at seven p.m. they were seated immediately and ordered their drinks and dinner.

During the course of the meals they consumed further quantities of wine.

It was a pleasant setting, and there was good-natured banter between the friends. They stayed at the restaurant until eight thirty p.m., during which a second bottle of wine was shared, while eating their meals. Later the waitress on seeing them completing their meal, fetched the bill and placed it on their table.

"The best thing about this restaurant is the chips," commented Angela.

And as Danielle placed a hand towards the waitress and breathed, "The best thing about this restaurant is you." Clearly, it was the alcohol 'talking.'

On leaving the restaurant, everyone appeared to be in a good mood and, as later understated by Angela Batley, "Nobody seemed too badly affected by alcohol, although we were fairly jolly."

The original plan was to drive from the restaurant to Angela and Harley's place, have a couple more drinks and further conversation. Oddly, Danielle drove her car back to her and Chiam's apartment, and Chiam went back to their friend's place. At the time it was thought that she was taking her dog Echo home, which was in the car. However, she later returned and still had the dog with her! The friends sat around and kept chatting. Danielle had some more red wine and Angela had some white wine. By the time it was to leave, after a "good couple of hours" Danielle appeared to be "getting a bit moody" and argumentative with Chiam.

Then he commented that, "It's lovely to be surrounded by happy, healthy people." After saying this, Danielle became sensitive about it, and said "What if we aren't healthy?" and that "it wasn't practical in everyday life."

The couple *apparently* left in Danielle's car.

## A Tumultuous Evening

Danielle walked in the front door at about eleven p.m. without the dog, and said to Jordan Kimel-August, Chiam's son: "I shouldn't have gone. I've had too much to drink."

She walked into the kitchen, put her handbag down and took out her iPod. Danielle later went to the living area of the apartment and started to play some music on a computer through the speakers of the computer. A short time later Chiam came into the room and asked her to turn down the volume because it would disturb the neighbours. She then turned it back up again. Jordan left the scene and went to his bedroom and shut the door.

Chiam then turned volume down again and Danielle kept turning the music up again. This occurred number times, and developed into an argument which became louder and more aggressive. Later Danielle was heard to say, "You fucking barred me out of the computer. You fucking barred me out of the computer"

Then as she proceeded to punch him, he said: "There's no need to get violent."

Things were now starting to get really out of hand, as she had now evidently reached for the antique knife on the coffee table and unsheathed it.

Seeing the knife, Chiam exclaimed, "What are you doing? Are you crazy?"

He then screamed in pain three times, as the knife was plunged into his body. Jordan opened his bedroom door to be confronted by an awful sight. His father had his left hand against the wall holding himself up and his right hand across his left ribcage. His white shirt was covered in blood.

He looked at his son and said, "She stabbed me. She stabbed me. Call the ambulance."

Danielle was standing opposite to Chiam holding the antique knife in her right hand. There was blood on her fingers. The sheaf, that the knife was normally kept in, was in her left hand.

She was crying as she said, "You fucking barred me out of the Internet."

When Jordan went back into his room to find a mobile phone, Danielle came into his room and said, "Get the fuck out. Get the fuck out."

At the same time she was indicating for Jordan to get out of the house while holding the knife.

Jordan said, "You fucking stabbed my father!"

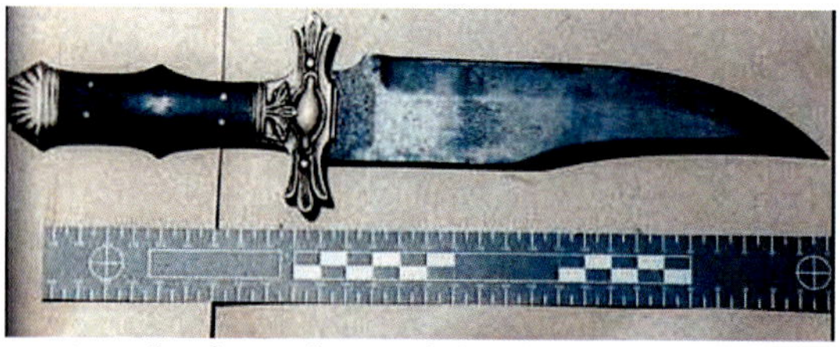

*Fig. 178. The antique knife used to stab her husband, Chaim Kimel to death. Photograph courtesy of NSW Police, Crime Scene.*

**A Dying Man**

Precious moments were ebbing away, and so was Chiam's life, as he was bleeding to death.

His son Jordan was desperate. He quickly put on some shorts and thongs and ran outside the apartment to the front door of a neighbour's home being the Mathew family. Jordan frantically knocked on the door and Josh Mathew answered the front door.

He then pleaded to him, "Please help. My father's been stabbed."

Josh, his brother Daniel and Jordan ran down the hall to help Chiam who was still lying in front of the elevator. There was blood everywhere.

Jordan then headed back down the hallway to get some more help from other neighbours. Just then, Danielle stormed out of the apartment holding the knife, the sheaf and a computer monitor.

Danielle then said loudly, "I stabbed him! I stabbed him! Look what he's done to me!"

She then dropped the computer flat screen monitor down where she was standing, and threw the bloodstained antique knife and its sheath down the stairs, and went back to the apartment.

In the meantime, Jordan went back to his father who was still on the mobile phone to an operator. The boys laid Chiam down in the elevator and took him to the ground floor.

"Call the ambulance. Call the ambulance," he kept saying.

Jordan then took the mobile off his father and spoke to the operator. He told them the address for the ambulance to come. This information was also passed onto the Police. Jordan was advised by the operator to get a clean cloth and put pressure on his father's wounds. Chiam was now in a bad way.

Jordan then placed a cushion under his head and he tried to calm him by saying, "Don't talk. Breathe deeply. Try not to move."

He said to his son, "I love you very much. Everything is going to be all right."

Jordan needed to go outside as the situation was becoming more than he could handle. He then became very angry, and ran into the laundry and grabbed a golf club. He ran out into the foyer brandishing the golf club and declaring, "I'm gonna kill her!"

Fortunately, Jordan was restrained by his friends, Josh and Daniel who calmed him down and told him "to be strong." Good advice. A very bad situation could have become decidedly worse.

The police then arrived. Jordan went back inside the building and sat by his father as the ambulance also arrived.

"Danielle…" gasped the dying man to the police, clutching a blood-soaked towel to his abdomen.

Chiam was loaded onto a stretcher and taken away to St Vincents Hospital for emergency surgery. Unfortunately, he died on the operating table that night, and it was now a case of murder.

The police went upstairs to find Danielle…

**'Study' Time**

It was easy to find Danielle Stewart. A thick trail of blood covering the carpet of the communal floor and splattering the walls, led police officers to the couple's front door apartment. On the way, Senior Constable Khaliph Fitzmaurice saw the antique knife with blood on its handle, at the bottom of the stairs in the common area of the building. The sheath for the knife lay nearby. Also observed was a computer flat screen on the stairs, splattered in blood, along with numerous receipts and various pieces of paperwork.

After getting no response to requests to open up, the police forced entry. On gaining entry to the Rose Bay Apartment, a curious sight befell them.

Danielle Stewart was sitting on a couch holding an iPod, notepad and pen.

One of the police officers, Sergeant Richard Lord asked Danielle Stewart, "Are you Danielle?"

To which she mimicked, "Are you Danielle?"

Sergeant Lord then took the iPod, pen and pad from Danielle and asked, "Where's the knife?"

She replied, "What knife?" and the added, "But I was studying!"

The police then explained her rights. Danielle Stewart then apparently quipped, "My rights, really? That's funny because you're in my house."

In the meantime, another police officer searched the apartment and found a blister pack of Seroquel tablets, a brand of quetiapine, under Ms Stewart's bed. Nineteen tablets were missing from the pack.

She was arrested and handcuffed. However, she refused to walk and so three police officers had to carry her to the police cage truck.

Danielle kicked and screamed all the way down to the police wagon, yelling out to her sixteen-year-old stepson (who fortunately, was not present): "How could you do this to me? After all I did for you! How could you betray me like this?!"

Once in the back of the wagon she lay motionless on the floor and bumps were heard each time the wagon turned the corner. Clearly, she was incapacitated and so it was fairly bumpy journey! However, due to her bizarre behaviour, which alternated between lucid to irrational, she was later transferred to an ambulance who took her to Prince of Wales Hospital to obtain blood samples. She was accompanied by Constable Julie-Anne Johnson.

On arrival at the hospital, Danielle Stewart turned and yelled at the police officer: "Bitch! Bitch!

She also abused doctors and nurses trying to calm her, "Don't you fucking touch me you bitch." She then fumed, "He wouldn't let me into the computer. He's taken all the money I put into my business. He's ruined my business. I want to call my grandmother. I have no mother or father, please let me call her, I don't have anyone."

Then strangely, she commented, "He's probably sitting at home fucking laughing at me."

Eventually, the blood samples were obtained and forwarded onto the Division of Analytical Laboratories at Lidcombe for analysis.

During the course of her treatment, Danielle was assessed both physically and psychologically. She was subsequently discharged from hospital at four p.m., and conveyed to Waverly Police Station where she was entered into custody and read her rights. Danielle Stewart was subsequently charged and, due to the circumstances, was taken into custody.

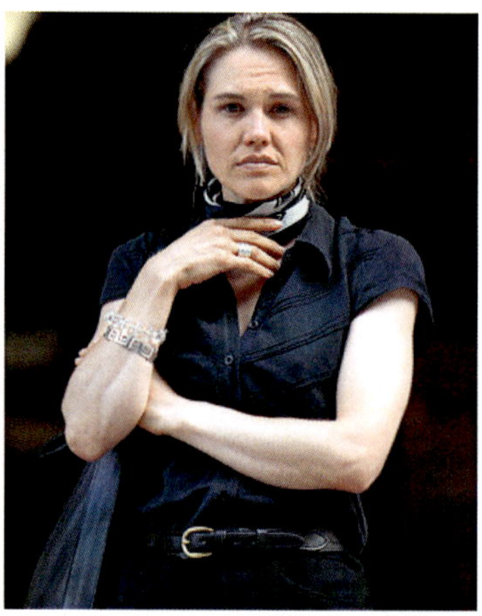

*Fig. 179. Danielle Stewart: Arrested over the stabbing of her husband, Chiam Kimel. Photograph courtesy of* The Daily Telegraph.

**On Trial for Murder**

On 7 July 2008, Daniel Stewart stood trial in the NSW Supreme Court at Taylor Square, Darlinghurst for the murder Chiam Kimel on the evening of the 23 August 2006.

A number of issues were raised during the trial, including Ms Stewart's personality disorder where she supposedly lived in constant fear that Mr Kimel would leave her. But, strangely, he also was considered "domineering, controlling in the relationship" and that she was "not strong enough to get away from him."

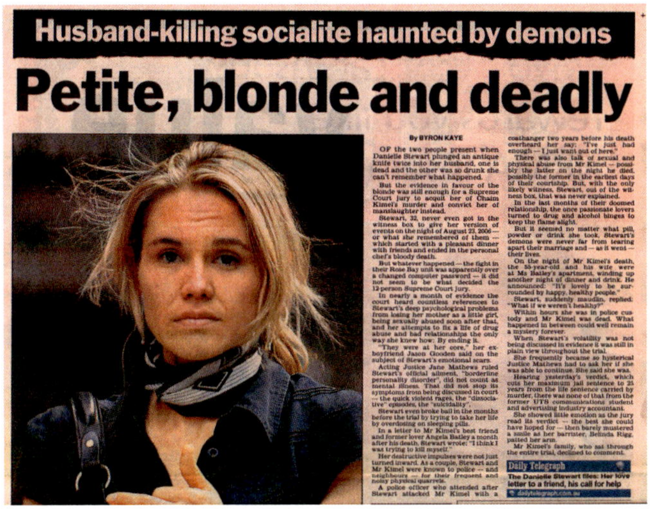

Husband-killing socialite haunted by demons

# Petite, blonde and deadly

By BYRON KAYE

OF the two people present when Danielle Stewart plunged an antique knife twice into her husband, one is dead and the other was so drunk she can't remember what happened.

But the evidence in favour of the blonde was still enough for a Supreme Court jury to acquit her of Chaim Kimel's murder and convict her of manslaughter instead.

Stewart, 32, never even got in the witness box to give her version of events on the night of August 23, 2006 — or what she remembered of them — which started with a pleasant dinner with friends and ended in the personal chef's bloody death.

But whatever happened — the fight in their Rose Bay unit was apparently over a changed computer password — it did not seem to be what decided the 12-person Supreme Court jury.

In nearly a month of evidence the court heard countless references to Stewart's deep psychological problems from losing her mother as a little girl, being sexually abused soon after that, and her attempts to fix a life of drug abuse and bad relationships the only way she knew how: By ending it.

"They were at her core," her ex-boyfriend Jason Gooden said on the subject of Stewart's emotional scars.

Acting Justice Jane Mathews ruled Stewart's official ailment, "borderline personality disorder", did not count as mental illness. That did not stop its symptoms from being discussed in court — the quick violent rages, the "dissociative" episodes, the "suicidality".

Stewart even broke bail in the months before the trial by trying to take her life by overdosing on sleeping pills.

In a letter to Mr Kimel's best friend and former lover Angela Batley a month after his death, Stewart wrote: "I think I was trying to kill myself."

Her destructive impulses were not just turned inward. As a couple, Stewart and Mr Kimel were known to police — and neighbours — for their frequent and noisy physical quarrels.

A police officer who attended after Stewart attacked Mr Kimel with a coathanger two years before his death overheard her say: "I've just had enough — I just want out of here."

There was also talk of sexual and physical abuse from Mr Kimel — possibly the latter on the night he died, possibly the former in the earliest days of their courtship. But, with the only likely witness, Stewart, out of the witness box, that was never explained.

In the last months of their doomed relationship, the once passionate lovers turned to drug and alcohol binges to keep the flame alight.

But it seemed no matter what pill, powder or drink she took, Stewart's demons were never far from tearing apart their marriage and — as it went — their lives.

On the night of Mr Kimel's death, the 55-year-old and his wife were at Ms Batley's apartment, winding up another night of dinner and drink. He announced: "It's lovely to be surrounded by happy, healthy people."

Stewart, suddenly maudlin, replied: "What if we weren't healthy?"

Within hours she was in police custody and Mr Kimel was dead. What happened in between could well remain a mystery forever.

When Stewart's volatility was not being discussed in evidence it was still in plain view throughout the trial.

She frequently became so hysterical Justice Mathews had to ask her if she was able to continue. She said she was.

Hearing yesterday's verdict, which cuts her maximum jail sentence to 25 years from the life sentence carried by murder, there was none of that from the former UTS communications student and advertising industry accountant.

She showed little emotion as the jury read its verdict — the best she could have hoped for — then barely mustered a smile as her barrister, Belinda Rigg, patted her arm.

Mr Kimel's family, who sat through the entire trial, declined to comment.

Daily Telegraph

The Danielle Stewart files: Her love letter to a friend, his call for help

dailytelegraph.com.au

*Fig. 180. The write up of Danielle Stewart: 'Petite, blonde and deadly' Courtesy of* The Daily Telegraph.

Poignantly, Ms Stewart's grandmother, Ms Elaine Kraker, was asked if the two loved each other, to which she replied: "Yes, and that's what I can't understand."

Tragically for Mr Kimel and his family, less than a month after murdering her husband with an antique knife, Danielle Stewart wrote to his best friend and former lover, Angela Batley, saying: "For really the first time in our relationship, everything was really good between Chiam and I." Adding, "Apart from a few hiccups we were closer to each other than we had ever been."

On page three of the letter she said:

"I'm so sorry, it should be me that's dead. I never meant to hurt Chiam, let alone kill him. There is not one single part of me that wants him dead. I want him alive. I want my life back. I want our life back."

It continued:

"He was my best friend. I have nothing without him. I woke one day with a beautiful life, then woke up 3 days later in hell." Further, "I am so traumatized knowing what this has done to his children. I love Jordan as if he was my own flesh and blood. I'm so worried that he doesn't have Chiam now, that he may have to live with Diana who doesn't give a shit about him really.

"Chiam was my whole life, as I know I was his whole life."

During the trial further revelations about their tumultuous relationship were revealed.

Dr Rosalind Foy was treating Ms Stewart for about five months before she fatally stabbed her husband with the antique knife.

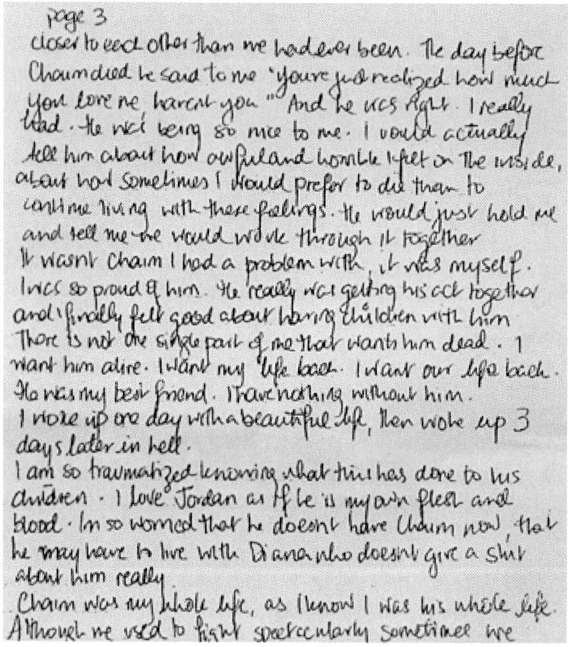

page 3
closer to each other than we had ever been. The day before
Chaim died he said to me "youre just realized how much
you love me, haven't you" And he was right. I really
had. He was being so nice to me. I would actually
tell him about how awful and horrible I felt on the inside,
about how sometimes I would prefer to die than to
continue living with these feelings. He would just hold me
and tell me we would work through it together
It wasn't Chaim I had a problem with, it was myself.
I was so proud of him. He really was getting his act together
and I finally felt good about having children with him
There is not one single part of me that wants him dead. I
want him alive. I want my life back. I want our life back.
He was my best friend. I have nothing without him.
I woke up one day with a beautiful life, then woke up 3
days later in hell.
I am so traumatized knowing what this has done to his
children. I love Jordan as if he is my own flesh and
blood. Im so worried that he doesnt have Chaim now, that
he may have to live with Diana who doesnt give a shit
about him really.
Chaim was my whole life, as I know I was his whole life.
Although we used to fight spectacularly sometimes we

*Fig. 181. A part letter of regret from the accused killer, Danielle Stewart's letter to her husband's best friend.*
*Source:* The Daily Telegraph.

She told the Supreme Court jury at Taylor Square that Ms Stewart suffered from a borderline personality disorder, similar to a post-traumatic stress disorder, as a result of being sexually abused by a number of people as a child.

Dr Foy described Ms Stewart as "deeply disturbed in an angry fashion" and had a "high level of anxiety."

But it was not just her childhood trauma that was raised, but an abortion two weeks earlier that left her "depressed and suicidal," continued Dr Foy.

"It was a very distressing thing for her," she said.

However, the pregnancy was not due to Mr Kimel, her husband!

Ms Stewart had become pregnant from another lover, whose name was given as Yuri Moel, when she had visited in Melbourne during a brief separation from Mr Kimel during 2005.

Further, Dr Foy told the Court: “Yuri had wanted to keep it [the child] and have her live with him in Melbourne. Chiam said have a termination if you want to stay with him.

“Danielle decided it was not the time to be having children.”

Ms Stewart’s barrister, Belinda Rigg suggested that Mr Kimel was “dominating and controlling and she’d get defensive and angry and they’d fight.”

Ms Stewart said that on the night of the stabbing she was acting in self-defence and that her husband had been physically violent towards her.

However, this was at odds with the evidence presented by Dr Foy who denied Ms Stewart had mentioned physical abuse at the hands of Mr Kimel during their lengthy sessions.

Dr Foy said, “She had difficulties with his personality. She would say she wasn’t happy with him. She was feeling isolated. They didn’t socialise very much and they didn’t have common friends except Angela [Bately] who was always miserable and who was an ex-partner of her husband.”

Further evidence was presented by Mr Kimel’s daughter, Mrs Amber Rubenstein. She told the Court that her father was a “gentle giant” who had been abused by Ms Stewart. Ms Stewart apparently had bitten him on the thumb and arm a number of times, and had smashed or damaged his glasses.

[A damaged set of glasses was found in the apartment on the night of the stabbing.]

Mrs Rubenstein said, “It became a running joke in the family that he had to get his glasses replaced regularly,” she continued, “When she became aggressive she would grab them and step on them, mangle them, I don’t know.”

Mrs Rubenstein further told the Court, “I saw her in happy moods. She was lovely, actually. I really liked her until I had seen, for myself, her aggressive outbursts.”

Mrs Rubenstein and her brother Fred Kimel also told how they faced the painful task of cleaning out the home that their father shared with Ms Stewart, only to come across a draft of a play written by Ms Stewart about a woman who plots her husband’s violent murder.

Mrs Rubenstein tearfully told the Court:

“I couldn’t believe my eyes, I was horrified and tormented by these revelations. After reading her writings I felt cheated – I didn’t know she had thoughts like this.

“There is a synopsis of a play in which one of the characters has secret desires to kill her husband in a violent rage,” she continued, “There are study notes on gaol architecture, prisoner psychology, different cell classifications, prison attire, prison visiting hours and life sentences.”

Fred Kimel commented, “How am I able to understand how someone could have perpetrated such a crime having already considered the potential ramifications?”

However, the unfinished manuscript was not allowed as evidence in the trial because there was uncertainty as to Ms Stewart’s sobriety, whether due to drugs and/or alcohol, at the time of writing.

A number of other witnesses came forward and gave evidence in relation to this matter, including myself. I was there to interpret the levels of drugs and alcohol found in Ms Stewart's blood and so determine how much she would have been affected at the time of the incident. Analysts' reports were supplied by the Analytical Laboratories of Lidcombe, New South Wales and by the Victorian Institute of Forensic Medicine, Southbank in Victoria. These agreed that she had the following levels of drugs and alcohol in her blood:

- diazepam 0.06-0.08 milligrams per litre,
- nordiazepam <0.01 milligrams per litre,
- temazepam <0.01 milligrams per litre.

But more important were the levels of drug, quetiapine and alcohol present in her blood:

- quetiapine 1.3 milligrams per litre, and
- alcohol 0.203 grams per decilitre (100 millilitres) of blood.

Quetiapine is available under the trade name of Seroquel ( but also known as AstraZeneca) and it is an antipsychotic drug which has been shown to be effective in the treatment of schizophrenia. Ms Stewart had indicated earlier that on the evening of the incident, she had taken "nearly the whole packet" of Seroquel on the evening of the incident, crushing some of the tablets into soya milk before drinking them. Whilst the level of quetiapine detected was significant, at just over double the top end of therapeutic range, the major player here was – alcohol.

I estimated that the level of alcohol in her blood at the time of the incident most likely at 0.240% and concluded that, "given the estimated blood alcohol level and the elevated level of quetiapine present in Ms Stewart's blood at the time of the incident, her ability to think rationally about her actions would have been compromised." A similar estimation of her blood alcohol at the time of the incident was confirmed by other experts involved in this matter. Dr Graham Starmer further described the alcohol level at the time of the incident as "swamping" the effects of the other drugs.

## The Verdict and Sentence

A jury by a majority verdict found that Daniel Stewart was not guilty of murdering her husband, but guilty of his manslaughter.

Ms Stewart said she was acting in self-defence when she stabbed Chiam Kimel in the stomach with an antique knife. However, the prosecution contended that there "was no element of self-defence in her actions", arguing she stabbed her husband in an argument over their catering business.

On December 16 2008 Acting Justice Jane Mathews, in sentencing Danielle Stewart, made reference to her blood alcohol reading at the time of the stabbing which was calculated to have been 0.240. The judge concluded that the combination of a high level of alcohol intoxication and Ms Stewart's borderline personality disorder led to the tragedy. Justice Mathews commented to Mr Kimel's three children seated in the public gallery:

"I suspect that you'll regard the punishment that that I am about to impose as quite inadequate to the extent of your loss."

However, she said that no punishment would ever be able to redress their loss and that there a number of factors to consider before delivering the sentence.

Justice Mathews then sentenced Ms Stewart to a maximum of six years and four months with a minimum of four years gaol, with the sentence backdated to when she was taken into custody.

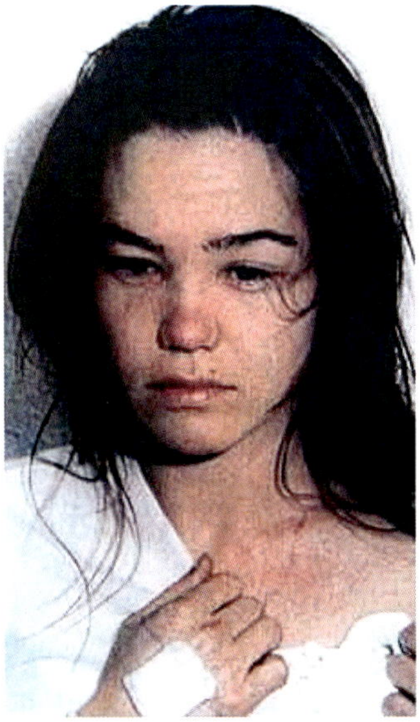

*Fig. 182. Danielle Stewart, after taken into custody.*
*No longer, 'Petite, blonde and – deadly' (maybe).*

By the time Danielle Stewart is released, she will have received appropriate treatment for her borderline personality disorder and, hopefully, also given up the alcohol. Otherwise, Fred Kimel's comment, "I worry that if she is not able to take full responsibility for her actions [that] she will always present a threat" may well become a prophecy.

Hopefully, this will not happen.

# Acknowledgements, Reference and Further Reading

**Chapter 1.**
My laboratory notes taken at the time, and my trusty trusty ol' high school inorganic chemistry text titled *Mellor's Modern Inorganic Chemistry*, G.D. Parkes (Editor), 1961, pp. 842-843 *['Arsenic for Dinner?']*

**Chapter 2.**
Assistance from Tamworth and Uralla Police (NSW) is gratefully acknowledged for the preparation of this story. *['A Cry in the Night']*

**Chapter 3.**
Assistance from New South Wales Police – Crime Scene, Sydney Police Centre, is gratefully acknowledged for this preparation of this story, which also appeared in the *Australian Police Journal* March 2005, Vol 59, No. 1 pp. 44-47. *['A Case of MDMA Madness']*

**Chapter 4.**
Assistance from New South Wales Police – Crime Scene, Sydney Police Centre, is gratefully acknowledged for this preparation of this story, which also appeared in the *Australian Police Journal* September 2005, Vol 59, No. 3 pp. 141-143. *['Affairs of the Heart and Poisons']*

**Chapter 5.**
Assistance from Wollongong Police (NSW) in particular, Sergeant Gregory Moon is gratefully acknowledged for supplying the facts and images involved this story. I must also acknowledge the *Illawarra Mercury* and Dr Alan Cala, a forensic pathologist, for extracts from his examination report of Liam's body as well as Detective Sergeant Barry Fay (retired) for the final edit which also appeared in the *Australian Police Journal* September 2012, Vol 66, No. 3 pp. 100-107. *['The Corpse in the Culvert']*

**Chapter 6.**
Assistance from Chatswood Police and Detective Sergeant V. A. Crawford in particular, is gratefully acknowledged for this story. *['No Laughing Matter']*

**Chapter 7.**
Assistance from the following people, Ms Barbara Barnes (DPP), and Detective Senior Constable Gavin Bradbury are gratefully acknowledged for the preparation of this article. *['Cuppa Anyone?']*

**Chapter 8.**
Assistance from the following people, Ms. Natalie Olender (DPP), Detective Senior Constable Kieran Beaumont, officer in charge of this matter at the time now at NSW State Crime Command's Unsolved Homicide Team, Detective Sergeant Kevin Sullivan (Bass Hill Crime Scene Section) and Detective Senior Constable Paul Arnold

(Auburn Detectives) are gratefully acknowledged for the preparation of this article which also appeared in the *Australian Police Journal* September 2008, Vol 62, No. 3 pp. 140-144 *['Steroids made me do it!']*

**Chapter 9.**
Assistance from the following Police officers, Senior Constable Sharyn Moiriarty (NSW Police Crime Scene), Field Co-ordinator, Andrew Brady (NSW Police Crime Scene) and Detective Sergeant Phil Dyball (Redfern Detectives) is gratefully acknowledged for the preparation of this story, which also appeared in the *Australian Police Journal* March 2006, Vol 60, No. 1 pp. 43-47 *['The Body in the Bin Murder']*

**Chapter 10.**
My sincere gratitude is expressed to the following police officers, Senior Constable Ken Cropper, Senior Constable O'Neill, Detective Senior Constable Donna Garten and Detective Sergeant Ed Freeman (now retired) for this story. Also, to Dr Malcolm Dodd, forensic pathologist, for extracts from his examination of Hudson's body. which also appeared in the *Australian Police Journal* June 2009, Vol 63, No. 2 pp. 84-87 *['Death of a Drug Dealer']*

**Chapter 11.**
My sincere gratitude is expressed to the Gunnedah Police (NSW) for the preparation of this story. *['Suicide on the Farm']*

**Chapter 12.**
My sincere gratitude is expressed to the following police officer, Detective Senior Constable Jenny Ross and also, to Dr Dianne Little, forensic pathologist, for extracts from her examination of deceased's body. *['Up in Smoke']*

**Chapter 13.**
My sincere gratitude is expressed to the City Central Local Area Command, Criminal Investigations and in particular, Detective Sergeant Kay Whitty, City Central Police Station and *The Daily Telegraph. ["Drink Spiking: A Two Man 'Crime Wave'."]* which also appeared in the *Australian Police Journal* December 2009, Vol 63, No. 4 pp. 164-167

**Chapter 14.**
Assistance from the following police officers, Detective Senior Constable Lindsay Kerfoot, Sergeant Matt Fordham, Senior Constable Bradley Helson and Dr Judy Perl is gratefully acknowledged. *['Methadone Mothers']* These cases were presented at "Methadone Mothers" 51$^{th}$ Meeting & Conference of The International Association of Forensic Toxicologists (TIAFT) Funchal, Portugal, September 2 – 6, 2013.

**Chapter 15.**
My sincere gratitude is expressed to the following police officers, Detective Senior Constable 'Gez' Green and Detective Senior Constable 'George' (Anasta) Georgopoulos, Burwood Detectives, NSW. *['The Case of the One-Armed Would-Be Rapist.']*

**Chapter 16.**
Assistance from the following police officers, Detective Senior Constable Eric Andrew (Leichhardt Detectives) and Detective Sergeant Matthew Schibeci, (Sydney Crime Scene Section) is gratefully acknowledged. *['The Lady in the Bath Water']*
This case was presented as *"A Propofol Assisted Death"* at 48th Meeting of The International Association of Forensic Toxicologists (TIAFT) Bonn, Germany. August 28 – 3 September (2010)

**Chapter 17.**
My sincere gratitude is expressed to the following police officers, Detective Senior Constable Matthew Harmer, Detective Senior Constable Scott Lawson of North Shore Police and Sergeant Brian Barns, Forensic Imaging, Sydney Police Centre, Surry Hills. *['The "Cheese Ball" Killer – The Car as a Murder Weapon']* This case was presented at the International Conference on Alcohol, Drugs and Traffic Safety, (ICADTS) Brisbane, Australia, (2013) August 25- 28

**Chapter 18.**
My sincere gratitude is expressed to the following police officers: Detective Senior Constable Benjamin Tearne, Rose Bay Detectives and Detective Senior Constable Gavin Bradbury, Kings Cross Detectives.*["Dr Suresh Nair – Cocaine Killer"]*

**Chapter 19.**
My sincere gratitude is expressed to the following police officer: Detective Sergeant Stephen Pollard, North Sydney Detectives. *["Death of a Dancer"]*

**Chapter 20.** Assistance from the following police officers, Detective Benjamin Tearne and Detective Sergeant Samuel Crisafulli, of Rose Bay is gratefully acknowledged. *["The Antique Knife"]*

# References and Further Reading

**Chapter 1.**
*Mellor's Modern Inorganic Chemistry*, G. D. Parkes (Editor), 1961, pp. 842-843.

**Chapter 2.**
MIMS 2000 re. 'Serepax' (oxazepam); *Isolation and Identification of Drugs in pharmaceuticals, body fluids and post-mortem material*, (1974) Volume 1, E. G. C. Clarke (Editor), Pharmaceutical Press, London p. 458.

**Chapter 3.**
Downing, J. (1986) J. *Psychoactive Drugs* 18: 335-340.

Greer, G. & Tolbert, R. (1986) J. *Psychoactive Drugs* 18: 319-328.

McGuire, P. & Fahy, T. (1991) *British Medical Journal* 302: 697.

O'Connor, B. (1994) Brit. J. Hosp. Med. 52(10): 507-514.

Solowij, N. Hall, W. & Lee, N. (1992) British Journal of Addiction. 87: 1161-1172.

NSW *Police Service Weekly* (2001) 13(14): 6.

Henry, J. A; Jeffreys, K. J. & Dawling, S. (1992) *The Lancet* 340: 384-387.

McKenna, D. J. & Peroutka, S. J. (1990) J. Neurochem. 54(1): 14-22.

**Chapter 4.**
*Pesticide Manual – A World Compendium* (1983) 7th Ed. The British Crop Protection Council (Eds), Lavenham Press (Publishers) pages: 5540, 8590.

**Chapter 5.**
Martindale – *The Extra Pharmacopoeia* 32nd Edition; LSD50.

**Chapter 6.**
Rosenberg, F. K. et al. (1979) *Annals of Cardiac Anaesthetics* 58: 104-106.

Wagner, S. A.; Wesche, M. A. & Clarke et al (1992) *Journal of Forensic Science*, 37: 1008-1015.

**Chapter 7.**
Martindale – *The Extra Pharmacopoeia* 32nd Edition; 'Hypnodorm' Flunitrazepam.

**Chapter 8.**
Martindale – *The Extra Pharmacopoeia* 32nd Edition; Steroids, Testrosterone "Anabolic Steroids – Ultimate Research Guide" (2005) Vol. 1 Anthony Roberts & Brian Clapp.

**Chapter 9.**
NIDA [National Institute on Drug Abuse] pamphlet: 'Heroin'.

**Chapter 10.**
Downing, J. (1986) *Journal of Psychoactive Drugs* 18: 335-340.

Greer, G. & Tolbert, R. (1986) *Journal of Psychoactive Drugs* 18: 319-328.

McGuire, P. & Fahy, T. (1991) *British Medical Journal* 302: 697.

O'Connor, B. (1994) *British Journal of Hospital Medicine.* 52(10): 507-514.

Solowij, N. Hall, W. & Lee, N. (1992) *British Journal of Addiction.* 87: 1161-1172.

NSW *Police Service Weekly* (2001) 13(14): 6.

Henry, J. A; Jeffreys, K. J. & Dawling, S. (1992) *The Lancet* 340: 384-387.

McKenna, D. J. & Peroutka, S. J. (1990) J. Neurochem. 54(1): 14-22.

**Chapter 11.**
*Arsenic poisoning – "Poisoning: Toxicology, Symptoms, Treatments"* (1986) 5th Ed. J. M. Arena & R. H. Drew (Eds) C. Thomas (Publisher), USA.

**Chapter 12.**
Huestis, M.; Henningfield, J. & Cone, E. (1992) *Journal of Analytical Toxicology.* 16 (5): 283-290.

Chiang, C. & Barnett, G. (1984) *Clinical Pharmacology*. Thera. 36 (2): 234-238; "Poisoning: Toxicology, Symptoms, Treatments" (1986) 5th Ed. J. M. Arena & R. H. Drew (Eds) C. Thomas (Publisher), USA.

**Chapter 13.**
*Drug facilitated Sexual Assault – A Forensic Handbook (2000)* M. A. LeBeau & A. Mozayani (Eds) Academic Press, pp. 97, 216.

**Chapter 14.**
*The Australian Drug Guide* Dr Jonathan Upfal (2000) 5th Edition Bookman Publishers, Australia pp. 425-428.

*Disposition of Toxic Drugs and Chemicals in Man* (2004) 7th Edition, Randall C. Baselt (Editor), Biomedical Publications, Foster City, California.

Wilson, P; Watson, R; & Ralston, G. E. (1994) Methadone maintenance in general practice: patients, workload, and outcomes. *British Medical Journal* 309: 641-644.

*MIMS* issue no. 3 (2000) p.413.

Clarke, J. C.; Milroy, C. M. & Forrest, A. R. W. (1995) Deaths from methadone use. *Journal of Clinical Forensic Medicine* 2: 143-144.

Binchy, J. M; Molyneux, E. M. & Manning, J. (1994) "Accidental ingestion of methadone by children in Merseyside" *British Medical Journal* 308: 1335-1336.

Arnow, R; Sashi, P. D. & Woolley, P. V. (1972) "Childhood poisoning: An unfortunate consequence of methadone availability." *Journal of the American Medical Association* 219: 321-324.

Smailek, J. E.; Monforte, J. R.; Aronow, R. & Spitz, W. U. (1977) "Methadone deaths in children: a continuing problem" *Journal of the American Medical Association.* 238: 2516-2517.

B. Geraghty, E. A. Graham, B. Logan & E. L. Weiss (1997) "Methadone levels in breast milk." *Journal of Human Lactation* 13(3): 227-230.

R. E. Wojnar-Horton, J. H. Kristensen, P. Yapp et al (1997) "Methadone distribution and excretion into breast milk of clients in a methadone maintenance programme." *British Journal of Clinical Pharmacology* 44(6): 543-547.

J. J. McCarthy & B. L. Posey (2000) "Methadone levels in human milk." *Journal of Human Lactation* 16(2): 115-120.

**Chapter 15.**

Norberg, A; Jones, W. A; Hahn, R. G. & Gabrielsson, J. L. (2003) "Role of variability in explaining ethanol pharmacokinetics." *Clinical Pharmacokinetics,* 42 (1): 1-31.

**Chapter 16.**

Iwersen-Bergmann, S; Rosner, P; Kuknau, H. C. Junge, M. & Schmoldt, A. (2001) 'Death after excessive propofol abuse.' *International Journal of Legal Medicine* 114: 248-251.

Hunter, D. D; Thornily, A; Whitburn, R. (1987) 'Arousal from propofol' *Anaethesiology* 77: 817-818.

Follette, J. W. & Farley, W.J. (1992) 'Anesthesiologist addicted to propofol' *Anesthesiology* 77: 817-818;

Fritz, G. A. & Niemczyk,W.E. (2002) 'Propofol dependency in a lay person.' *Anesthesiology* 96: 505-506.

Canaday, B. R. (1993) 'Drug Experience: Amorous, disinhibited behaviour associated with propofol' *Clinical Pharmacy* 12: 449-451.

Drummer, O.H.(1992) 'A fatality due to propofol poisoning.' *Journal of Forensic Sciences* 37(4): 1186-1189.

**Chapter 17.**

*Winek's Drug & Chemical Blood-Level Data 2001* Charles L. Winek (Editor).

*Disposition of Toxic Drugs and Chemicals in Man* (2004) Randall C. Baselt (Ed) 7th Edition, Biomedical Publications, California.

**Chapter 18.**

*Sydney Morning Herald,* 2010-2011.

*The Daily Telegraph,* 2009.

*The Age,* 2009.

*The Australian*, December, 2010.

*Disposition of Toxic Drugs and Chemicals in Man* (2004) Randall C. Baselt (Ed) 7th Edition, Biomedical Publications, California, pp 256-262.

*Winek's Drug & Chemical Blood-Level Data 2001* Charles L. Winek (Editor).

**Chapter 19**

*Bulletin of The International Association of Forensic Toxicologists* (1996) Vol. 26 No. 1 Supplement.

*Disposition of Toxic Drugs and Chemicals in Man* Randall C. Baselt (Ed) 7th Edition, Biomedical Publications, California, pp 706-707.

**Chapter 20**

Norberg, A; Jones, W. A; Hahn, R. G. & Gabrielsson, J. L. (2003) "Role of variability in explaining ethanol pharmacokinetics." *Clinical Pharmacokinetics* 42 (1): 1-31.